# ACCESS YOUR ONLINE RESOURCES

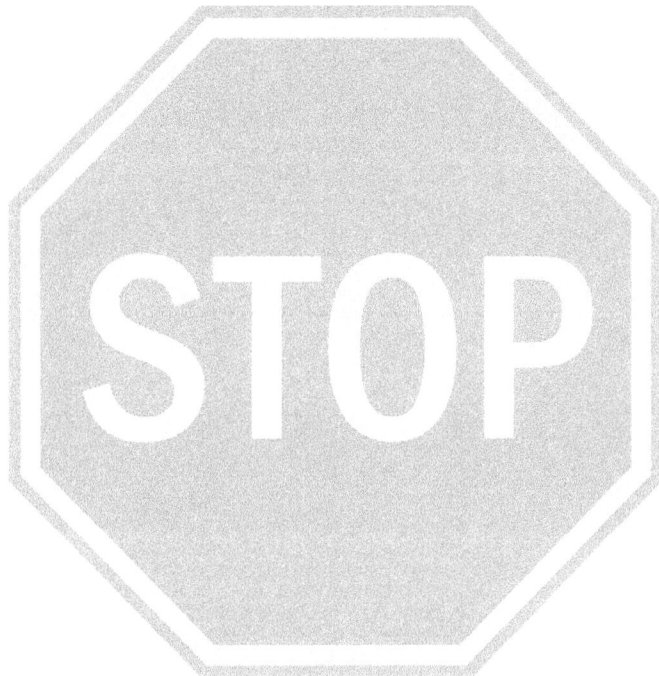

**DON'T MISS OUT ON THE ONLINE RESOURCES INCLUDED WITH YOUR PURCHASE!**

Your purchase of this product unlocks access to our Online Resources page. Elevate your study experience with our **interactive practice test interface**, along with all of the additional resources that we couldn't include in this book.

**Flip to the Online Resources section at the end of this book to find the link and a QR code to get started!**

# M✓metrix

## TEST PREPARATION

# NCTRC®
# Exam Secrets
# Study Guide

**NCTRC® Test Review for the National Council for Therapeutic Recreation Certification Exam**

# Mometrix
## TEST PREPARATION

Written and edited by the Mometrix Recreational Therapy Certification Test Team

Mometrix offers volume discount pricing to institutions. For more information or a price quote, please contact our sales department at sales@mometrix.com or 888-248-1219.

NCTRC and National Council for Therapeutic Recreation Certification are registered trademarks of National Council for Therapeutic Recreation Certification, Inc., which is not affiliated with Mometrix Test Preparation and does not endorse this product.

Paperback
ISBN 13: 978-1-61072-246-9
ISBN 10: 1-61072-246-9

Ebook
ISBN 13: 978-1-62120-434-3
ISBN 10: 1-62120-434-0

Hardback
ISBN 13: 978-1-5167-0812-3
ISBN 10: 1-5167-0812-1

# Dear Future Exam Success Story

First of all, **THANK YOU** for purchasing Mometrix study materials!

Second, congratulations! You are one of the few determined test-takers who are committed to doing whatever it takes to excel on your exam. **You have come to the right place.** We developed these study materials with one goal in mind: to deliver you the information you need in a format that's concise and easy to use.

In addition to optimizing your guide for the content of the test, we've outlined our recommended steps for breaking down the preparation process into small, attainable goals so you can make sure you stay on track.

We've also analyzed the entire test-taking process, identifying the most common pitfalls and showing how you can overcome them and be ready for any curveball the test throws you.

Standardized testing is one of the biggest obstacles on your road to success, which only increases the importance of doing well in the high-pressure, high-stakes environment of test day. Your results on this test could have a significant impact on your future, and this guide provides the information and practical advice to help you achieve your full potential on test day.

### Your success is our success

**We would love to hear from you!** If you would like to share the story of your exam success or if you have any questions or comments in regard to our products, please contact us at **800-673-8175** or **support@mometrix.com**.

Thanks again for your business and we wish you continued success!

Sincerely,
The Mometrix Test Preparation Team

---

**Need more help? Check out our flashcards at:**
**http://mometrixflashcards.com/NCTRC**

# TABLE OF CONTENTS

# Introduction

**Thank you for purchasing this resource!** You have made the choice to prepare yourself for a test that could have a huge impact on your future, and this guide is designed to help you be fully ready for test day. Obviously, it's important to have a solid understanding of the test material, but you also need to be prepared for the unique environment and stressors of the test, so that you can perform to the best of your abilities.

For this purpose, the first section that appears in this guide is the **Secret Keys**. We've devoted countless hours to meticulously researching what works and what doesn't, and we've boiled down our findings to the five most impactful steps you can take to improve your performance on the test. We start at the beginning with study planning and move through the preparation process, all the way to the testing strategies that will help you get the most out of what you know when you're finally sitting in front of the test.

We recommend that you start preparing for your test as far in advance as possible. However, if you've bought this guide as a last-minute study resource and only have a few days before your test, we recommend that you skip over the first two Secret Keys since they address a long-term study plan.

If you struggle with **test anxiety**, we strongly encourage you to check out our recommendations for how you can overcome it. Test anxiety is a formidable foe, but it can be beaten, and we want to make sure you have the tools you need to defeat it.

# Secret Key #1 – Plan Big, Study Small

There's a lot riding on your performance. If you want to ace this test, you're going to need to keep your skills sharp and the material fresh in your mind. You need a plan that lets you review everything you need to know while still fitting in your schedule. We'll break this strategy down into three categories.

## Information Organization

Start with the information you already have: the official test outline. From this, you can make a complete list of all the concepts you need to cover before the test. Organize these concepts into groups that can be studied together, and create a list of any related vocabulary you need to learn so you can brush up on any difficult terms. You'll want to keep this vocabulary list handy once you actually start studying since you may need to add to it along the way.

## Time Management

Once you have your set of study concepts, decide how to spread them out over the time you have left before the test. Break your study plan into small, clear goals so you have a manageable task for each day and know exactly what you're doing. Then just focus on one small step at a time. When you manage your time this way, you don't need to spend hours at a time studying. Studying a small block of content for a short period each day helps you retain information better and avoid stressing over how much you have left to do. You can relax knowing that you have a plan to cover everything in time. In order for this strategy to be effective though, you have to start studying early and stick to your schedule. Avoid the exhaustion and futility that comes from last-minute cramming!

## Study Environment

The environment you study in has a big impact on your learning. Studying in a coffee shop, while probably more enjoyable, is not likely to be as fruitful as studying in a quiet room. It's important to keep distractions to a minimum. You're only planning to study for a short block of time, so make the most of it. Don't pause to check your phone or get up to find a snack. It's also important to **avoid multitasking**. Research has consistently shown that multitasking will make your studying dramatically less effective. Your study area should also be comfortable and well-lit so you don't have the distraction of straining your eyes or sitting on an uncomfortable chair.

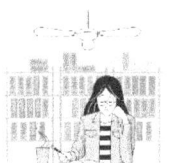

The time of day you study is also important. You want to be rested and alert. Don't wait until just before bedtime. Study when you'll be most likely to comprehend and remember. Even better, if you know what time of day your test will be, set that time aside for study. That way your brain will be used to working on that subject at that specific time and you'll have a better chance of recalling information.

Finally, it can be helpful to team up with others who are studying for the same test. Your actual studying should be done in as isolated an environment as possible, but the work of organizing the information and setting up the study plan can be divided up. In between study sessions, you can discuss with your teammates the concepts that you're all studying and quiz each other on the details. Just be sure that your teammates are as serious about the test as you are. If you find that your study time is being replaced with social time, you might need to find a new team.

2

# Secret Key #2 – Make Your Studying Count

You're devoting a lot of time and effort to preparing for this test, so you want to be absolutely certain it will pay off. This means doing more than just reading the content and hoping you can remember it on test day. It's important to make every minute of study count. There are two main areas you can focus on to make your studying count.

## Retention

It doesn't matter how much time you study if you can't remember the material. You need to make sure you are retaining the concepts. To check your retention of the information you're learning, try recalling it at later times with minimal prompting. Try carrying around flashcards and glance at one or two from time to time or ask a friend who's also studying for the test to quiz you.

To enhance your retention, look for ways to put the information into practice so that you can apply it rather than simply recalling it. If you're using the information in practical ways, it will be much easier to remember. Similarly, it helps to solidify a concept in your mind if you're not only reading it to yourself but also explaining it to someone else. Ask a friend to let you teach them about a concept you're a little shaky on (or speak aloud to an imaginary audience if necessary). As you try to summarize, define, give examples, and answer your friend's questions, you'll understand the concepts better and they will stay with you longer. Finally, step back for a big picture view and ask yourself how each piece of information fits with the whole subject. When you link the different concepts together and see them working together as a whole, it's easier to remember the individual components.

Finally, practice showing your work on any multi-step problems, even if you're just studying. Writing out each step you take to solve a problem will help solidify the process in your mind, and you'll be more likely to remember it during the test.

## Modality

*Modality* simply refers to the means or method by which you study. Choosing a study modality that fits your own individual learning style is crucial. No two people learn best in exactly the same way, so it's important to know your strengths and use them to your advantage.

For example, if you learn best by visualization, focus on visualizing a concept in your mind and draw an image or a diagram. Try color-coding your notes, illustrating them, or creating symbols that will trigger your mind to recall a learned concept. If you learn best by hearing or discussing information, find a study partner who learns the same way or read aloud to yourself. Think about how to put the information in your own words. Imagine that you are giving a lecture on the topic and record yourself so you can listen to it later.

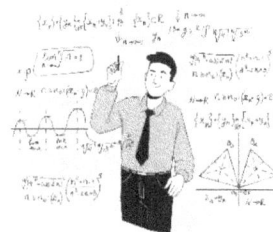

For any learning style, flashcards can be helpful. Organize the information so you can take advantage of spare moments to review. Underline key words or phrases. Use different colors for different categories. Mnemonic devices (such as creating a short list in which every item starts with the same letter) can also help with retention. Find what works best for you and use it to store the information in your mind most effectively and easily.

# Secret Key #3 – Practice the Right Way

Your success on test day depends not only on how many hours you put into preparing, but also on whether you prepared the right way. It's good to check along the way to see if your studying is paying off. One of the most effective ways to do this is by taking practice tests to evaluate your progress. Practice tests are useful because they show exactly where you need to improve. Every time you take a practice test, pay special attention to these three groups of questions:

- The questions you got wrong
- The questions you had to guess on, even if you guessed right
- The questions you found difficult or slow to work through

This will show you exactly what your weak areas are, and where you need to devote more study time. Ask yourself why each of these questions gave you trouble. Was it because you didn't understand the material? Was it because you didn't remember the vocabulary? Do you need more repetitions on this type of question to build speed and confidence? Dig into those questions and figure out how you can strengthen your weak areas as you go back to review the material.

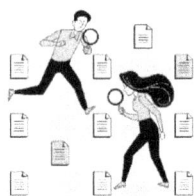

Additionally, many practice tests have a section explaining the answer choices. It can be tempting to read the explanation and think that you now have a good understanding of the concept. However, an explanation likely only covers part of the question's broader context. Even if the explanation makes perfect sense, **go back and investigate** every concept related to the question until you're positive you have a thorough understanding.

As you go along, keep in mind that the practice test is just that: practice. Memorizing these questions and answers will not be very helpful on the actual test because it is unlikely to have any of the same exact questions. If you only know the right answers to the sample questions, you won't be prepared for the real thing. **Study the concepts** until you understand them fully, and then you'll be able to answer any question that shows up on the test.

It's important to wait on the practice tests until you're ready. If you take a test on your first day of study, you may be overwhelmed by the amount of material covered and how much you need to learn. Work up to it gradually.

On test day, you'll need to be prepared for answering questions, managing your time, and using the test-taking strategies you've learned. It's a lot to balance, like a mental marathon that will have a big impact on your future. Like training for a marathon, you'll need to start slowly and work your way up. When test day arrives, you'll be ready.

Start with the strategies you've read in the first two Secret Keys—plan your course and study in the way that works best for you. If you have time, consider using multiple study resources to get different approaches to the same concepts. It can be helpful to see difficult concepts from more than one angle. Then find a good source for practice tests. Many times, the test website will suggest potential study resources or provide sample tests.

4

# Practice Test Strategy

If you're able to find at least three practice tests, we recommend this strategy:

## UNTIMED AND OPEN-BOOK PRACTICE

Take the first test with no time constraints and with your notes and study guide handy. Take your time and focus on applying the strategies you've learned.

## TIMED AND OPEN-BOOK PRACTICE

Take the second practice test open-book as well, but set a timer and practice pacing yourself to finish in time.

## TIMED AND CLOSED-BOOK PRACTICE

Take any other practice tests as if it were test day. Set a timer and put away your study materials. Sit at a table or desk in a quiet room, imagine yourself at the testing center, and answer questions as quickly and accurately as possible.

Keep repeating timed and closed-book tests on a regular basis until you run out of practice tests or it's time for the actual test. Your mind will be ready for the schedule and stress of test day, and you'll be able to focus on recalling the material you've learned.

# Secret Key #4 – Pace Yourself

Once you're fully prepared for the material on the test, your biggest challenge on test day will be managing your time. Just knowing that the clock is ticking can make you panic even if you have plenty of time left. Work on pacing yourself so you can build confidence against the time constraints of the exam. Pacing is a difficult skill to master, especially in a high-pressure environment, so **practice is vital**.

Set time expectations for your pace based on how much time is available. For example, if a section has 60 questions and the time limit is 30 minutes, you know you have to average 30 seconds or less per question in order to answer them all. Although 30 seconds is the hard limit, set 25 seconds per question as your goal, so you reserve extra time to spend on harder questions. When you budget extra time for the harder questions, you no longer have any reason to stress when those questions take longer to answer.

Don't let this time expectation distract you from working through the test at a calm, steady pace, but keep it in mind so you don't spend too much time on any one question. Recognize that taking extra time on one question you don't understand may keep you from answering two that you do understand later in the test. If your time limit for a question is up and you're still not sure of the answer, mark it and move on, and come back to it later if the time and the test format allow. If the testing format doesn't allow you to return to earlier questions, just make an educated guess; then put it out of your mind and move on.

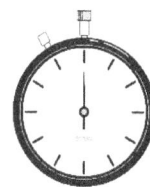

On the easier questions, be careful not to rush. It may seem wise to hurry through them so you have more time for the challenging ones, but it's not worth missing one if you know the concept and just didn't take the time to read the question fully. Work efficiently but make sure you understand the question and have looked at all of the answer choices, since more than one may seem right at first.

Even if you're paying attention to the time, you may find yourself a little behind at some point. You should speed up to get back on track, but do so wisely. Don't panic; just take a few seconds less on each question until you're caught up. Don't guess without thinking, but do look through the answer choices and eliminate any you know are wrong. If you can get down to two choices, it is often worthwhile to guess from those. Once you've chosen an answer, move on and don't dwell on any that you skipped or had to hurry through. If a question was taking too long, chances are it was one of the harder ones, so you weren't as likely to get it right anyway.

On the other hand, if you find yourself getting ahead of schedule, it may be beneficial to slow down a little. The more quickly you work, the more likely you are to make a careless mistake that will affect your score. You've budgeted time for each question, so don't be afraid to spend that time. Practice an efficient but careful pace to get the most out of the time you have.

# Secret Key #5 – Have a Plan for Guessing

When you're taking the test, you may find yourself stuck on a question. Some of the answer choices seem better than others, but you don't see the one answer choice that is obviously correct. What do you do?

The scenario described above is very common, yet most test takers have not effectively prepared for it. Developing and practicing a plan for guessing may be one of the single most effective uses of your time as you get ready for the exam.

In developing your plan for guessing, there are three questions to address:

- When should you start the guessing process?
- How should you narrow down the choices?
- Which answer should you choose?

## When to Start the Guessing Process

Unless your plan for guessing is to select C every time (which, despite its merits, is not what we recommend), you need to leave yourself enough time to apply your answer elimination strategies. Since you have a limited amount of time for each question, that means that if you're going to give yourself the best shot at guessing correctly, you have to decide quickly whether or not you will guess.

Of course, the best-case scenario is that you don't have to guess at all, so first, see if you can answer the question based on your knowledge of the subject and basic reasoning skills. Focus on the key words in the question and try to jog your memory of related topics. Give yourself a chance to bring the knowledge to mind, but once you realize that you don't have (or you can't access) the knowledge you need to answer the question, it's time to start the guessing process.

It's almost always better to start the guessing process too early than too late. It only takes a few seconds to remember something and answer the question from knowledge. Carefully eliminating wrong answer choices takes longer. Plus, going through the process of eliminating answer choices can actually help jog your memory.

**Summary**: Start the guessing process as soon as you decide that you can't answer the question based on your knowledge.

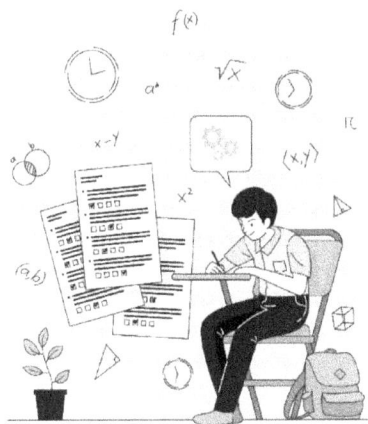

7

# How to Narrow Down the Choices

The next chapter in this book (**Test-Taking Strategies**) includes a wide range of strategies for how to approach questions and how to look for answer choices to eliminate. You will definitely want to read those carefully, practice them, and figure out which ones work best for you. Here though, we're going to address a mindset rather than a particular strategy.

Your odds of guessing an answer correctly depend on how many options you are choosing from.

| Number of options left | 5 | 4 | 3 | 2 | 1 |
|---|---|---|---|---|---|
| Odds of guessing correctly | 20% | 25% | 33% | 50% | 100% |

You can see from this chart just how valuable it is to be able to eliminate incorrect answers and make an educated guess, but there are two things that many test takers do that cause them to miss out on the benefits of guessing:

- Accidentally eliminating the correct answer
- Selecting an answer based on an impression

We'll look at the first one here, and the second one in the next section.

To avoid accidentally eliminating the correct answer, we recommend a thought exercise called **the $5 challenge**. In this challenge, you only eliminate an answer choice from contention if you are willing to bet $5 on it being wrong. Why $5? Five dollars is a small but not insignificant amount of money. It's an amount you could afford to lose but wouldn't want to throw away. And while losing $5 once might not hurt too much, doing it twenty times will set you back $100. In the same way, each small decision you make—eliminating a choice here, guessing on a question there—won't by itself impact your score very much, but when you put them all together, they can make a big difference. By holding each answer choice elimination decision to a higher standard, you can reduce the risk of accidentally eliminating the correct answer.

The $5 challenge can also be applied in a positive sense: If you are willing to bet $5 that an answer choice *is* correct, go ahead and mark it as correct.

**Summary**: Only eliminate an answer choice if you are willing to bet $5 that it is wrong.

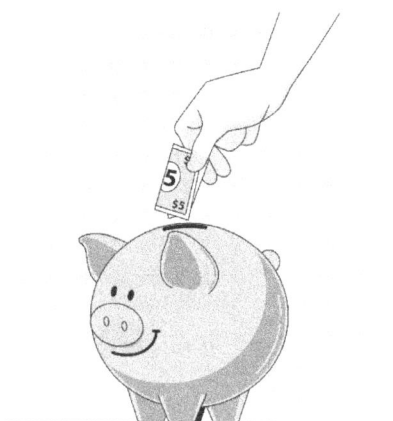

8

# Which Answer to Choose

You're taking the test. You've run into a hard question and decided you'll have to guess. You've eliminated all the answer choices you're willing to bet $5 on. Now you have to pick an answer. Why do we even need to talk about this? Why can't you just pick whichever one you feel like when the time comes?

The answer to these questions is that if you don't come into the test with a plan, you'll rely on your impression to select an answer choice, and if you do that, you risk falling into a trap. The test writers know that everyone who takes their test will be guessing on some of the questions, so they intentionally write wrong answer choices to seem plausible. You still have to pick an answer though, and if the wrong answer choices are designed to look right, how can you ever be sure that you're not falling for their trap? The best solution we've found to this dilemma is to take the decision out of your hands entirely. Here is the process we recommend:

**Once you've eliminated any choices that you are confident (willing to bet $5) are wrong, select the first remaining choice as your answer.**

Whether you choose to select the first remaining choice, the second, or the last, the important thing is that you use some preselected standard. Using this approach guarantees that you will not be enticed into selecting an answer choice that looks right, because you are not basing your decision on how the answer choices look.

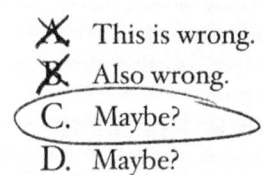

~~A.~~ This is wrong.
~~B.~~ Also wrong.
C. Maybe?
D. Maybe?

This is not meant to make you question your knowledge. Instead, it is to help you recognize the difference between your knowledge and your impressions. There's a huge difference between thinking an answer is right because of what you know, and thinking an answer is right because it looks or sounds like it should be right.

**Summary**: To ensure that your selection is appropriately random, make a predetermined selection from among all answer choices you have not eliminated.

9

# Test-Taking Strategies

This section contains a list of test-taking strategies that you may find helpful as you work through the test. By taking what you know and applying logical thought, you can maximize your chances of answering any question correctly!

It is very important to realize that every question is different and every person is different: no single strategy will work on every question, and no single strategy will work for every person. That's why we've included all of them here, so you can try them out and determine which ones work best for different types of questions and which ones work best for you.

## Question Strategies

### ⊘ READ CAREFULLY

Read the question and the answer choices carefully. Don't miss the question because you misread the terms. You have plenty of time to read each question thoroughly and make sure you understand what is being asked. Yet a happy medium must be attained, so don't waste too much time. You must read carefully and efficiently.

### ⊘ CONTEXTUAL CLUES

Look for contextual clues. If the question includes a word you are not familiar with, look at the immediate context for some indication of what the word might mean. Contextual clues can often give you all the information you need to decipher the meaning of an unfamiliar word. Even if you can't determine the meaning, you may be able to narrow down the possibilities enough to make a solid guess at the answer to the question.

### ⊘ PREFIXES

If you're having trouble with a word in the question or answer choices, try dissecting it. Take advantage of every clue that the word might include. Prefixes can be a huge help. Usually, they allow you to determine a basic meaning. *Pre-* means before, *post-* means after, *pro-* is positive, *de-* is negative. From prefixes, you can get an idea of the general meaning of the word and try to put it into context.

### ⊘ HEDGE WORDS

Watch out for critical hedge words, such as *likely, may, can, often, almost, mostly, usually, generally, rarely,* and *sometimes.* Question writers insert these hedge phrases to cover every possibility. Often an answer choice will be wrong simply because it leaves no room for exception. Be on guard for answer choices that have definitive words such as *exactly* and *always.*

### ⊘ SWITCHBACK WORDS

Stay alert for *switchbacks.* These are the words and phrases frequently used to alert you to shifts in thought. The most common switchback words are *but, although,* and *however.* Others include *nevertheless, on the other hand, even though, while, in spite of, despite,* and *regardless of.* Switchback words are important to catch because they can change the direction of the question or an answer choice.

## ⊘ Face Value

When in doubt, use common sense. Accept the situation in the problem at face value. Don't read too much into it. These problems will not require you to make wild assumptions. If you have to go beyond creativity and warp time or space in order to have an answer choice fit the question, then you should move on and consider the other answer choices. These are normal problems rooted in reality. The applicable relationship or explanation may not be readily apparent, but it is there for you to figure out. Use your common sense to interpret anything that isn't clear.

# Answer Choice Strategies

## ⊘ Answer Selection

The most thorough way to pick an answer choice is to identify and eliminate wrong answers until only one is left, then confirm it is the correct answer. Sometimes an answer choice may immediately seem right, but be careful. The test writers will usually put more than one reasonable answer choice on each question, so take a second to read all of them and make sure that the other choices are not equally obvious. As long as you have time left, it is better to read every answer choice than to pick the first one that looks right without checking the others.

## ⊘ Answer Choice Families

An answer choice family consists of two (in rare cases, three) answer choices that are very similar in construction and cannot all be true at the same time. If you see two answer choices that are direct opposites or parallels, one of them is usually the correct answer. For instance, if one answer choice says that quantity $x$ increases and another either says that quantity $x$ decreases (opposite) or says that quantity $y$ increases (parallel), then those answer choices would fall into the same family. An answer choice that doesn't match the construction of the answer choice family is more likely to be incorrect. Most questions will not have answer choice families, but when they do appear, you should be prepared to recognize them.

## ⊘ Eliminate Answers

Eliminate answer choices as soon as you realize they are wrong, but make sure you consider all possibilities. If you are eliminating answer choices and realize that the last one you are left with is also wrong, don't panic. Start over and consider each choice again. There may be something you missed the first time that you will realize on the second pass.

## ⊘ Avoid Fact Traps

Don't be distracted by an answer choice that is factually true but doesn't answer the question. You are looking for the choice that answers the question. Stay focused on what the question is asking for so you don't accidentally pick an answer that is true but incorrect. Always go back to the question and make sure the answer choice you've selected actually answers the question and is not merely a true statement.

## ⊘ Extreme Statements

In general, you should avoid answers that put forth extreme actions as standard practice or proclaim controversial ideas as established fact. An answer choice that states the "process should be used in certain situations, if…" is much more likely to be correct than one that states the "process should be discontinued completely." The first is a calm rational statement and doesn't even make a definitive, uncompromising stance, using a hedge word *if* to provide wiggle room, whereas the second choice is far more extreme.

11

### ⊘ Benchmark

As you read through the answer choices and you come across one that seems to answer the question well, mentally select that answer choice. This is not your final answer, but it's the one that will help you evaluate the other answer choices. The one that you selected is your benchmark or standard for judging each of the other answer choices. Every other answer choice must be compared to your benchmark. That choice is correct until proven otherwise by another answer choice beating it. If you find a better answer, then that one becomes your new benchmark. Once you've decided that no other choice answers the question as well as your benchmark, you have your final answer.

### ⊘ Predict the Answer

Before you even start looking at the answer choices, it is often best to try to predict the answer. When you come up with the answer on your own, it is easier to avoid distractions and traps because you will know exactly what to look for. The right answer choice is unlikely to be word-for-word what you came up with, but it should be a close match. Even if you are confident that you have the right answer, you should still take the time to read each option before moving on.

## General Strategies

### ⊘ Tough Questions

If you are stumped on a problem or it appears too hard or too difficult, don't waste time. Move on! Remember though, if you can quickly check for obviously incorrect answer choices, your chances of guessing correctly are greatly improved. Before you completely give up, at least try to knock out a couple of possible answers. Eliminate what you can and then guess at the remaining answer choices before moving on.

### ⊘ Check Your Work

Since you will probably not know every term listed and the answer to every question, it is important that you get credit for the ones that you do know. Don't miss any questions through careless mistakes. If at all possible, try to take a second to look back over your answer selection and make sure you've selected the correct answer choice and haven't made a costly careless mistake (such as marking an answer choice that you didn't mean to mark). This quick double check should more than pay for itself in caught mistakes for the time it costs.

### ⊘ Pace Yourself

It's easy to be overwhelmed when you're looking at a page full of questions; your mind is confused and full of random thoughts, and the clock is ticking down faster than you would like. Calm down and maintain the pace that you have set for yourself. Especially as you get down to the last few minutes of the test, don't let the small numbers on the clock make you panic. As long as you are on track by monitoring your pace, you are guaranteed to have time for each question.

### ⊘ Don't Rush

It is very easy to make errors when you are in a hurry. Maintaining a fast pace in answering questions is pointless if it makes you miss questions that you would have gotten right otherwise. Test writers like to include distracting information and wrong answers that seem right. Taking a little extra time to avoid careless mistakes can make all the difference in your test score. Find a pace that allows you to be confident in the answers that you select.

12

## ⊘ Keep Moving

Panicking will not help you pass the test, so do your best to stay calm and keep moving. Taking deep breaths and going through the answer elimination steps you practiced can help to break through a stress barrier and keep your pace.

# Final Notes

The combination of a solid foundation of content knowledge and the confidence that comes from practicing your plan for applying that knowledge is the key to maximizing your performance on test day. As your foundation of content knowledge is built up and strengthened, you'll find that the strategies included in this chapter become more and more effective in helping you quickly sift through the distractions and traps of the test to isolate the correct answer.

Now that you're preparing to move forward into the test content chapters of this book, be sure to keep your goal in mind. As you read, think about how you will be able to apply this information on the test. If you've already seen sample questions for the test and you have an idea of the question format and style, try to come up with questions of your own that you can answer based on what you're reading. This will give you valuable practice applying your knowledge in the same ways you can expect to on test day.

**Good luck and good studying!**

# Professionalism

## Develop Professional Relationships

### HISTORY OF RECREATIONAL THERAPY
#### HISTORICAL INFLUENCES IN THE 19TH AND 20TH CENTURIES

Before industrialization, doctors made house calls to wealthy people and hospitals charitably treated poor people. During and after the industrial revolution in the 19th century, hospitals transformed to educational and practice centers for physicians. As healthcare emphasis shifted to research, more people with disabilities/disorders were institutionalized. Social reform brought more state institutions and more humane care before World War I, though institutions still segregated people with disabilities. However, increases in public and private agencies serving them enabled new professions to develop, including TR/RT as well as PT, OT, etc. Additional effects of the industrial revolution included miserable urban conditions with pollution, poverty, and children unsupervised by either parents working long factory hours or schools, leading to juvenile delinquency. The establishment of the YMCA, with many local branches, provided recreational opportunities and social reform, education, youth work, and athletic leadership, revitalizing cities. Another improvement addressing urban blight was the playground movement, giving children places to socialize and play appropriately. The Playground Association of America (PAA) was formed (1906). The National Education Association identified leisure as necessary (1918), developing the first leisure education programs. The PAA became the National Recreation Association (1930), providing one of TR/RT's professional foundations.

#### EVOLUTION OF PHILOSOPHICAL ORIENTATIONS AND PROFESSIONAL ORGANIZATIONS

The TR/RT field originally evolved with two distinct philosophical perspectives:

- **Hospital recreation** emphasized the profession's role and value of offering meaningful recreational experiences and opportunities affording enjoyment/pleasure
- **Recreation therapy** emphasized using recreational activities therapeutically to remediate/treat specific disabilities/illnesses.

Leadership from the 1960s on made these ideological positions less separate, eventually uniting them under the name Therapeutic Recreation. In addition to the American Recreation Society (ARS, 1948), Hospital Recreation Section (HRS, 1949), RT Section (1952) of the American Association for Health, Physical Education, Recreation, and Dance (AAHPERD), and National Association of Recreational Therapists (NART, 1953), the **National Therapeutic Recreation Society** (1966–2010) was a prominent professional organization unifying recreational therapists. The field worked for decades to achieve recognition as a distinct health and human services profession through a respected knowledge base, ethical codes, professional practice standards, acknowledged educational and training programs, formally organized members, and service to society. Despite the profession's maturity, recent healthcare and other social changes demand continual adaptations. The **American Therapeutic Recreation Association** (ATRA) formed in 1984, reinforcing TR/RT's healthcare position. Diverse populations, settings, roles, and responsibilities are addressed by standards of certification, licensure, and accreditation.

#### SIGNIFICANT DEVELOPMENTS IN THE 1980S-1990S

The National Therapeutic Recreation Society (NTRS, 1966–2010) was a branch of the National Recreation and Park Association (NRPA). During the 1980s, the NTRS Registration Board was

15

separated from the NRPA. This was because the National Organization for Competency Assurance (National Commission for Health Certifying Agencies until 1987, renamed Institute for Credentialing Excellence [ICE] in 2009) made recognition of the NTRS Registration Board's certification plan contingent upon the board's independence from NRPA. Also, during the 1980s, ATRA members collaborated with the Joint Commission and CARF International to incorporate the Standards of Practice of TR Service into their review processes. NCTRC took on the establishment, administration, and management of standards for certifying and recertifying TR/RT professionals. To enhance its credentialing program, NCTRC began its Job Analysis Project in 1987, using curriculum and practitioner studies to define the required entry-level TR/RT knowledge base. Findings confirmed professional consensus that it needed stability and consistency to enable creating a national certification examination, among other things. NCTRC contracted with Educational Testing Service (ETS) to develop a 200-item written test, first available in 1990. Also in 1990, NRPA contractor Applied Measurement Professionals published a leisure professional certification exam including TR items.

## EVOLUTION OF RECREATIONAL THERAPY AS A VEHICLE FOR EXPERIENCING RECREATION

TR/RT has not been viewed and used only as a therapeutic tool, but also as a vehicle for experiencing recreation. In the early 20th century, some agencies for the blind and special schools for children with developmental disabilities started offering camping and other recreational programs for the children they served for the purposes of providing opportunities for normal enjoyment and fun, as well as rehabilitation and training. Special educators advised parents, teachers, and administrators that by playing games, children were not only playing, but receiving training that developed their attention, coordination, self-control, patience, manners, altruism, morals, and numerous additional positive skills, and socialized them. 1972 research showed participation in play activities enabled children with developmental disabilities to adjust better to their living circumstances emotionally and socially. The American Red Cross initiated early uses of recreation for hospitalized patients, particularly wounded soldiers in VA hospitals, followed by state mental hospitals, alleviating boredom and behavior problems, and then specialty hospitals. Thus, the therapeutic use of recreation reciprocally made therapy a recreative process.

## PARTNERING WITH HIGHER EDUCATION TO ADVANCE THE PROFESSION

After the Therapeutic Recreation Education Conference (TREC) in 2005 and again in 2009, which met to improve the professional preparation programs of higher education institutions for prospective TRSs, the Council on Accreditation of Parks, Recreation, Tourism, and Related Professions (COAPRT) developed a strategic plan for making TR/RT accreditation criteria compliant with the recommendations of the Council for Higher Education Accreditation (CHEA) of focusing on transparent, accountable management processes and measures of outcomes. This plan led to revision of the standards and operational procedures for the educational preparation of undergraduate and graduate TR/RT students and for professional TR/RT accreditation. These revisions became effective in 2013. While it still existed in 2009, the NTRS signed an affiliate agreement with COAPRT to establish student results for accrediting TR/RT as a specialty profession. ATRA's publication, *Guidelines for Competency Assessment and Curriculum Planning for Recreational Therapy Practice* (2008), inspired TR/RT professionals to explore alternatives for accreditation, including reinforcing professional education/preparation programs by aligning with healthcare organizations. ATRA was accepted in 2010 as a sponsoring member of educational programs for TR/RT practice by The Commission on Accreditation of Allied Health Programs (CAAHP), recognizing the Committee on Accreditation of Recreational Therapy Education (CARTE) as the accrediting body.

## INTERDISCIPLINARY TEAMWORK

Performance improvement in the workplace has placed significant emphasis on using teams and on self-management by teams. With quality improvement and safety being top priorities of management, they find that forming teams for improving care and coming up with solutions is a critical practice. TRSs will often be members of such teams. This includes not only **interdisciplinary service teams** and **department or unit teams,** but also **quality improvement teams**, on which they may serve along with managers as well as other service and other staff members. As team members, their responsibilities can vary. By working together, professionals can access the strength of the group and the collective knowledge and expertise of its members. To be effective team members, TRSs need skills including collaboration skills, group processing skills, individual accountability, positive interdependence, face-to-face interaction skills, communication skills, trust, cooperation, problem-solving skills, and conflict resolution skills. They must understand team dynamics. TRSs may work with physicians, nurses, physical therapists, occupational therapists, speech-language pathologists, audiologists, psychologists, counselors, social workers, educational specialists, teachers, clergy, correctional personnel, and other disciplines depending on the individual client, program, agency, and setting.

### COLLABORATION WITH HEALTH AND HUMAN SERVICE PROFESSIONALS

Health and human service professions that collaborate with the RT through co-treatment, consultation, and referral include:

- **Psychologist**: Evaluate, diagnose, and provide treatment for mental health and behavioral issues.
- **Speech therapist**: Evaluate and treat communication and swallowing disorders.
- **Occupational therapist**: Evaluate abilities and assist clients to manage activities of daily living, such as cooking, bathing, and other personal care and usual activities.
- **Physical therapist**: Evaluates and provides exercise regiments in order to improve or restore function, reduce discomfort, and prevent complications.
- **Social worker**: Evaluates, serves as case manager, makes referrals, identifies resources available to the client, educates, and assists with financial and housing needs.
- **Nurse**: Assesses and provides medical treatments.
- **Physician**: Prescribes treatments as appropriate for client needs.
- **Substance abuse counselor**: Evaluates, identifies needs, teaches coping mechanisms, leads group therapy, makes referrals to support groups or other community resources, assists with job planning, provides court reports regarding client's progress.

### COLLABORATING FOR CLIENTS WITH COMORBID MENTAL HEALTH AND SUBSTANCE ABUSE

Suppose an individual is diagnosed with comorbid mental health and substance abuse disorders. As often happens, this individual used substance(s) attempting to self-medicate mental illness symptoms, inadvertently causing dependency. A holistic health and human services model requires treating the whole person. Involved in this individual's treatment would be a physician addressing medical/health concerns; nurses assisting the physician and performing services not requiring an MD; a psychiatrist addressing the mental illness, which can include prescribing medication, consulting, and providing individual and/or group therapy and counseling; a psychologist specializing in substance abuse treatment and counseling; a support group leader; a rehabilitation program director, coordinator, and other staff; and a social worker providing social services and support because the client has been unable to secure/maintain employment due to mental illness symptoms and substance abuse effects, and from lack of funds may need help with housing, food, and aforementioned health services. The social worker may also coordinate these various services as case manager. Suppose also the psychologist and rehabilitation staff recommend TR/RT to replace substance abuse activities. TR/RT also addresses many mental health-related needs.

### COLLABORATING FOR CLIENTS WITH VISION OR HEARING IMPAIRMENT

Individuals with visual impairments typically receive services from orientation and mobility (O&M) specialists to teach them how to determine their locations/positions in buildings and outdoor areas away from home, navigate through unfamiliar surroundings, use canes, etc. Some people may also receive services from specialists who train seeing-eye dogs and teach clients how to work with their new service dogs. A TRS with a blind client would collaborate and coordinate with these professionals so the client can participate in leisure and recreational activities using the necessary O&M skills and integrating the dog's assistance. TRSs serving blind military veterans might also work with personnel from the Department of Veteran Affairs' Blind Rehabilitation Service or the Blinded Veterans Association; they may work with US Association of Blind Athletes and International Blind Sports Association personnel to help visually impaired athletes compete. TRSs serving deaf/hearing-impaired clients will frequently work with deaf educators, ASL interpreters, audiologists, hearing aid specialists, and personnel from the USA Deaf Sports Federation and/or International Committee of Sports for the Deaf which sponsors the Deaflympics, to help clients develop sports skills, participate, and compete.

# Maintain Professional Competency

### CLIENT ADVOCACY

Rapid, significant changes in society increasingly require TRSs to adopt roles as **advocates** for their clients. As the internet has enabled an explosion of accessible health and medical information, and medical science and technology have advanced, health care is becoming globalized, and the expectations of people, societies, and governments regarding disease prevention, health promotion, and personal care have risen. Even in isolated and developing areas, as innovations in technology, pharmacology, knowledge, and therapies become available, healthcare providers and recipients are accessing them. Changes are so rapid that their occurrence and people's experience of them are virtually simultaneous. More successful medical care, fewer acute and more chronic conditions, and aging populations are extending health care past treatment to such issues as global disease prevention, substance abuse, sexual predation, violence, and obesity. TRSs must network with varied healthcare, social service, community, and education agencies to deliver holistic, evidence-based, efficient care. In their roles as advocates, they must be accountable for client outcomes promoting positive lifestyle behaviors and health. TRSs promote health and prevent illness through active interventions using aerobic exercise, stress management, adventure/challenge, lifestyle awareness, physical fitness, coping skills, and patient health education.

> **Review Video: Patient Advocacy**
> Visit mometrix.com/academy and enter code: 202160

### HIPAA'S ROLE IN PROMOTING CLIENT ADVOCACY

The client has the right to complete or relative **confidentiality**. Only those with the need to know and with the consent of the client or client's agent can access client information. Exceptions include child, older adult, and persons with disabilities abuse (which must be reported to the appropriate authorities) and cases in which the client is a threat to self or others. Recreation therapists must comply with **HIPAA regulations** related to any health information as a client advocate:

- **Privacy rule**: Protected information includes information included in the medical record (electronic or paper), conversations between the doctor and other healthcare providers, billing information, and any other form of health information.
- **Security rule**: Electronic health information must be secure and protected against threats, hazards, or non-permitted disclosures. Administrative, physical, and technical safeguards must be in place as well as policies and procedures to comply with standards. Security requirements include: limiting access to those authorized, use of unique identifiers for each user, automatic logoff, encryption and decryption of protected healthcare information, authentication that healthcare data has not been altered/destroyed, monitoring of logins, authentication, and security of transmission. Access controls must include unique identifier, procedure to access system in emergencies, time out, and encryption/decryption.

> **Review Video: HIPAA**
> Visit mometrix.com/academy and enter code: 412009

## ADDRESSING CLIENT COMPLAINTS

Each organization should develop a formal **grievance policy** that includes the steps that the client should take if the client has a complaint. Policies may vary but often include the following:

- Directly address the complaint to the director of the program, who should respond by telephone or in person within a prescribed period of time, such as 24 to 48 hours.
- If the client does not feel that the director has satisfactorily resolved the problem, then the client should file a formal written complaint.
- The formal complaint should be presented in writing (a complaint form may be available) as directed to the director or board of directors within a prescribed period of time, such as within 30 days of the incident.
- The organization should carry out an investigation and fact-finding to determine the validity of the complaint and any steps that should be taken to remedy situations.
- The client should receive a formal response in writing within a prescribed period of time, such as 30 days.

## PROFESSIONAL ADVOCACY

TRSs not only advance their profession through marketing, they also survey and identify client needs and wants, service gaps, and develop services and products that clients and caregivers find relevant. By encouraging clients to develop long-term relationships with service providers, they advocate for their health maintenance and wellbeing. When TRSs improve cost-effectiveness, quality of care, service accessibility, and accomplish results that clients value more predictably and regularly, they provide value-added services, which health and human service organizations have found essential to their success. Value-added services ensure client satisfaction, which in turn promotes their staying in or returning to the same service network. Analyses of agency strengths, weaknesses, opportunities, and threats (SWOT) enable TR/RT agencies to respond proactively to stakeholder trends and influences; identify target markets, client needs and preferences, and agency capacities for meeting these; and design programs and evaluations to improve client functioning, health, and quality of life. TRSs also advocate by recruiting others as advocates.

## PUBLIC RELATIONS, PROMOTION, AND MARKETING

When TRSs develop marketing plans, they follow procedures similar to those they use during the assessment, planning, implementation, and evaluation (APIE) process. They identify internal resources (strengths and weaknesses) in their agencies and compare these to the external factors (opportunities and threats) in the surrounding environment, through SWOT analysis. Through such analysis, they discover the forces and developments that affect clients' functioning, health, and overall quality of life. They can then proactively design programs and evaluations to improve these, as well as identify their agency/department's target markets and their particular preferences and needs. They can also compare their agency's ability to meet these needs to the abilities of other agencies in the current competitive health and human services environment. During implementation, TRSs set schedules and choose the most appropriate methods for enlisting their target markets' support and then engage in the activities that will help them develop relationships with them.

## CULTURAL COMPETENCE

### ELEMENTS

Elements of competency for the RT include:

- **Cultural**: Awareness of different cultural practice and norms, willingness to incorporate cultural values into treatment plans, and respect for differences. Recognizing personal cultural ideals and biases. Recognizing and respecting proxemics in different cultures.
- **Educational**: Recognition of different styles of learning and assessment of readiness to learn and needs for learning. Willingness to alter methods to meet the client's needs and to encourage the client to actively engage in learning. Understanding the balance between skill and challenge.
- **Language**: Comprehension of cultural contexts of language and awareness of both verbal and nonverbal communication. Recognition of the need for translators or alternate methods of communication.
- **Environmental**: Awareness of different attitudes and needs toward environmental factors, such as housing, political attitudes, economic status, and physical needs, and the impact that environmental factors (climate, nutrition, household situation, temperature) have on a client's growth and development.

### INFLUENCE OF CULTURAL FACTORS ON TR/RT PROCESSES

In the APIE process, cultural influences are most vividly reflected in the assessment portion. Both assessment content and methods of data collection are influenced by cultural characteristics. For example, client culture determines whether and how clients make eye contact; their orientations to and attitudes toward space and time; communication styles; and their values, beliefs and opinions about autonomy, independence, health, and family roles. Culture also determines a client's background experiences with leisure and recreation, which in turn inform the TRS's choice of assessment instruments and data collection methods. In order to develop comprehensive databases on clients, TRSs will design or procure one or more techniques and tools for gathering information. They can select tools that are consistent with the types of services and programs they will offer by choosing assessment tools best suited to these. Available instruments are classified according to their main purposes and content, enabling the TRS to select the most compatible ones.

### BENEFITS OF CULTURAL SENSITIVITY IN RESPONSE TO DIVERSITY

As demographic changes are contributing to increasing diversity in America, and technology is also providing opportunities for people to communicate across geographic borders, health and human services are correspondingly becoming more diverse. To offer services to all populations, it is necessary to have a diverse workforce. Cultural sensitivity and support of diversity are becoming more common in managerial mission statements and resources that employers provide to their staffs. Both existing and new employees are receiving more preparation for performing competently in diverse environments, in the forms of cultural diversity integrated into coursework, workshops for professionals, and staff trainings. Today, entry-level practitioners are recommended to have specific competency in understanding one's own culture and its effects on and relationships with other cultural groups and understanding the impact of culture on clinical practice and communication. Professionals can augment their capacities for providing effective services by having or attaining awareness and sensitivity to different cultural perspectives. Hence multicultural competence not only affects productivity, but moreover increases employee retention in the workforce.

## HISTORY, ATTITUDES, STEREOTYPES, AND MYTHS SURROUNDING DISABILITY

Although in some instances persons with disabling conditions have experiences similar to those several decades ago, in many other ways their lives have changed dramatically in recent years. Since the Americans with Disabilities Act (ADA) was passed in 1990, people with disabilities are guaranteed the same civil rights protections previously promised to other minority populations. However, it must be remembered that the social reform that follows the passage of such a major act of law can take a great many years to be implemented and for all aspects of society to change in ways that reflect the legal mandates. All of the potential results of the law will also take a long time to be revealed. Attitudes toward groups and individuals are manifested in the imagery of popular culture. Traditionally these were called stereotypes, implying that they are inaccurate products of ignorance. Stereotypes are also fixed by definition: they do not change, but are abandoned once exposed as untrue and societies move beyond them. However, myths associated with disability are more deep-seated than stereotypes; sociologists call these constructions.

### ATTITUDES TOWARDS DISABILITY PROJECTED BY POPULAR CULTURE

The symbols and images produced by popular culture reflect societal attitudes; reciprocally, they also influence those attitudes. The ways in which disabilities are represented in our culture and society frequently reflect current ideas found in social management, science, medicine, and/or religion. However, these ideas themselves can also be influenced by the assumptions that are implicit in fictional narratives and popular cultural images. For example, a movie that depicts how a dedicated physician helps a child who has a disability to walk could very likely reflect the currently predominant approaches to disabilities of the medical profession in our society. As a publicly consumed art form, the movie disseminates medical and social attitudes toward disabilities, making an impression on the general public, people with disabilities, their families, and their caregivers. However, at the same time, practicing physicians would also be viewing the movie and others similar to it. Therefore, doctors would contribute to the cultural and social evidence whereby physicians perceive the status of their patients who have disabilities and their own status as medical practitioners.

### SOCIOLOGICAL CONSTRUCTIONS REGARDING PERCEPTIONS OF DISABILITY

What sociologists refer to as constructions are deeply rooted beliefs or conceptions, which represent ways of understanding and portraying a concept such as disability. In the late 1990s, experts studying the history of disability referred to six common constructions long used in society to organize human experience relative to the idea of disability (cf. *Beyond Affliction: The Disability History Project*). These constructions consisted of paired polar opposites:

- They express the same assumptions in both positive and negative forms.
- They are seldom observed in isolated, pure form; concepts, even those contradicting one another, frequently are combined/overlap in fictional/historical figures.
- They create long-term, culturally pervasive images of both power and ambiguity. Such constructions continue over generations and geographical borders.
- They sustain transformations.
- They disappear and re-emerge, existing covertly within ostensibly value-free, objective plans and analyses.
- They continue to influence the lives of persons with disabilities, their families, and service providers.

People with disabilities have sometimes resisted these constructions to define their own existences, at other times applied them. Constructions are not simplistically inaccurate, containing grains of truth. However, as implicit assumptions underlying social interactions and public policy, they restrict the complete humanity of the people involved.

## SIX COMMON SOCIAL CONSTRUCTIONS OF DISABILITY IN HUMAN SOCIETY

Six social constructions or deeply rooted beliefs or perceptions about disability have often been identified by historians and sociologists. They are composed in part of folklore, part of myth, and part of widespread societal attitudes. The **first three** constructions are as follows:

- The idea that people with disabilities are different from other human beings. They are viewed as lesser and "other," as limited or partial human beings. Because many people with disabilities are easily identified, this "other" status makes metaphors of them for the concept of experiencing alienation from society.
- Another construction is that people with disabilities who are successful in society and life are somehow superhuman. Their overcoming the obstacles and adversity they face makes them an example for others. They are seen as models of courage, patience, and persistence. Their disabilities become opportunities for them to demonstrate virtues, which they had never considered as virtues.
- A third construction is that disability represents a permanent, continual burden of suffering for nondisabled family/significant others. Nondisabled family/caregivers, always obligated to help them, are viewed as nobly sacrificing, inspiring others to benevolence and charity.

The **remaining three** social constructions regarding disability are the following:

- The idea that disability is abnormality/dysfunction/illness needing to be fixed/cured. Incurable disabilities, or those not responding to curative attempts, are viewed as tragic.
- People with disabilities are viewed as menaces to society, other people, and themselves—particularly those with intellectual disabilities, seen as lacking moral sense to avoid hurting themselves and others. People with disabilities are perceived as inevitably consumed by rage at the disability and nondisabled others.
- People with disabilities, particularly cognitive, are seen as "holy innocents" whose "special grace" inspires others, with extraordinary talents compensating for their other limitations.

## PERCEPTION OF DISABILITIES BY INDIVIDUALS WITH DISABILITIES

Common misconceptions about individuals with disabilities include the following:

- Disability defines individuals, or others label individuals by disability.
- People with disabilities are constantly ill/in pain (typically untrue).
- People with disabilities are courageous/inspirational. They find such expectations, not their disabilities, burdensome
- People with disabilities should be treated differently as "special." This undermines equality.
- Disability is a personal tragedy/burden. Disability does not dictate poor quality of life; negative societal attitudes and community lack of accessibility do.
- People with disabilities always need help/are dependent. They may/may not; nondisabled people should not assume they do, but ask.
- People with disabilities only want to interact socially with others having disabilities. Friendships and relationships are personal choices and preferences. Not all people with disabilities, even with similar characteristics, want to associate/be friends with one another.
- People in wheelchairs are "confined" to them. This is analogous to seeing ambulatory people as "confined" to their automobiles. People using wheelchairs view them like cars, as forms of mobility supporting independence.
- People with disabilities are one-dimensional, with the same needs/interests/opinions. Actually, they reflect society's diversity/individual differences.
- People with disabilities cannot lead productive, full community lives. They can, when abilities, not limitations, are the focus.

# CREDENTIALING

## DEVELOPMENT OF NATIONAL AND STATE CREDENTIALLING

The **Commission for the Advancement of Hospital Recreation (CAHR)** originally developed a national credentialing or registration plan for TRSs in 1956. In 1969, the National Therapeutic Recreation Society (NTRS) made significant modifications in this plan to reflect the changes that had since transpired in TRS education and training, and trends in current TR/RT practice. One of these modifications was to appoint the Continuing Professional Development Review Board, whose task was to review and endorse the constantly growing array of TR/RT training opportunities that offered the greatest benefits to the profession's educational needs. At the state level, during the late 1960s and early 1970s, initial efforts produced Recreation Therapy Practice Acts, which licensed therapists in Georgia and Utah. Although Georgia was unable to maintain this Practice Act, since 1975 Utah has continued to offer state licensure. Since then, Washington, D.C., New Hampshire, North Carolina, and Oklahoma require state licensure for TRSs. New York and Pennsylvania are seeking licensure. California and Washington State have title protection acts for TRSs.

## NATIONAL COUNCIL FOR THERAPEUTIC RECREATION CERTIFICATION (NCTRC)
### VISION, MISSION, AND GOALS

The **National Council for Therapeutic Recreation Certification (NCTRC) is** a national and international nonprofit organization providing the Certified Therapeutic Recreation Specialist (CTRS) credential promoting professional excellence for consumer protection. Formed in 1981, NCTRC is recognized by the Commission for Accreditation of Rehabilitation Facilities (CARF) and the Joint Commission. It is a charter member of the Institute of Credentialing Excellence (ICE) and accredited by the National Commission for Certifying Agencies (NCCA). NCTRC's vision includes public recognition as the largest international CTRS body; primary consumer, employer, and regulator recognition; research and technology use to improve its critical functions and certification examination program; promotion of the credential's value and validity; effective, viable organizational marketing; TR/RT credentialing opportunity information provision; and research opportunity enhancement. NCTRC's mission is to protect TR/RT service consumers by furthering quality TR/RT service provision from CTRSs. NCTRC strategic goals include creating broadly based partnerships; creating certification across the global market; leading in consumer protection; developing innovative opportunities for practitioners, consumers, and policymakers in education, training, and research; and promoting the value of the CTRS credential.

## NCTRC CERTIFICATION ELIGIBILITY AND ACADEMIC PATH

Applicants must submit transcripts of a baccalaureate or higher degree majoring in TR, or in recreation or leisure with a TR option, from an accredited university/college. This includes at least 18 semester/24 quarter hours of TR and general recreation coursework; at least 15 semester/20 quarter hours of TR content; at least 5 TR courses, minimum 3 credit hours each. Recommended course content includes assessment, the TR process, and advancement of the profession. Required supportive courses totaling 18 semester/24 quarter hours must include at least 3 semester/4 quarter hours in anatomy and physiology; 3 semester/4 quarter hours in abnormal psychology; 3 semester/4 quarter hours in lifespan human growth and development, with the remainder in social sciences and humanities. The required TR/RT services field placement experience, using the NCTRC's current Job Analysis Study's definition of the TR process, is at least 14 consecutive weeks, 560 hours, supervised by both agency and academic supervisors with NCTRC CTRS credentials, following most coursework completion. Applicants enrolled in TR/RT degree programs can apply for professional eligibility reviews before completing their degrees after completing all coursework except field placement, and at least 90 credit hours toward the degree, and submitting official transcripts.

## INTERNSHIP OPPORTUNITIES

Students preparing to become TRSs are required to participate in substantial field experience in addition to completing academic coursework to be eligible to take NCTRC's examination, which they must pass to earn the CTRS credential. The American Therapeutic Recreation Association (ATRA), the main TR/RT professional organization, offers an excellent information resource in its extensive online internship database. (ATRA cautions users that opportunities listed do not necessarily meet NCTRC certification or state licensure standards, and to consult internship coordinators/academic advisors for choosing suitable placements.) Just a few examples include a TR Intern/Group Assistant position at The Autism Project, a private practice setting working with children and adolescents; a TR internship working with people of all ages having developmental and physical disabilities at a parks and recreation agency; a TR internship at a physical rehabilitation hospital unit, working with adults and older adults having physical disabilities; RT internship at a behavioral and mental health hospital unit, working with adults and older adults; RT internship working with a geriatric adult population in short-term rehabilitation programs at a long-term care facility; and a program internship in a community program, working with adolescents, adults, and older adults with developmental and physical disabilities.

## NCTRC EQUIVALENCY PATH

CTRS applicants **without the TR/RT field placement** required in the academic path defined by the NCTRC must complete the same 18 semester/24 quarter hours of TR and general recreation courses including at least 15 semester/20 quarter hours TR content, at least 5 TR courses, 3 hours minimum each. However, the applicant can have taught two of the three TR courses as a full-time educator. NCTRC recommendations for coursework in assessment, the TR process, and advancement of the profession are the same as for the academic path. Whereas NCTRC academic-path requirements are 18 semester/24 quarter hours, at least half divided among anatomy and physiology, abnormal psychology, lifespan human growth and development (at least 3 semester/4 quarter hours each) and the rest in social sciences and humanities; in equivalency paths, required supportive course hours are at least 24 semester/32 quarter hours, in any social sciences and humanities subjects, plus at least five years of paid full-time work experiences in TR services as NCTRC's current Job Analysis defines these; for applicants with graduate TR degrees, at least three years or the aforementioned 18/24 academic-path course content hours, plus at least one year of CTRS-supervised, paid, full-time TRS work experience.

## NCTRC RECERTIFICATION

NCTRC reviews and processes about 1,200 new applications annually for professional eligibility for Certified Therapeutic Recreation Specialist (CTRS) credentials. Graduates with academic majors/options in TR/RT, within 12 months of graduation, comprise around 95% of new applications. During the five-year certification cycle, CTRSs must submit annual maintenance applications and fees. CTRSs must recertify every five years. NCTRC offers two recertification options:

- **Continuing education credit** related to the NCTRC Job Analysis and professional work experience in TR/RT; OR
- A **passing score on the national certification examination**. Recertification applications must show the applicant has completed these continuing competence requirements and include annual maintenance fees.

CTRSs with extensive expertise and experience in specific areas of TR/RT practice may apply for NCTRC specialty certification. Expert skills, acquired successfully over substantial practice periods, education programs, and training focusing on specific diagnostic populations and/or skills contribute to advanced knowledge and skills attained. Specialty certification intends to acknowledge advanced professional levels of CTRS practice and formally recognize competence beyond the basic credential. The NCTRC national standardized certification examination and continuous credential verification and monitoring services are additional NCTRC services provided.

## PROFESSIONAL DEVELOPMENT

Experts note that effective organizations in the 21st century are viewed as "learning organizations" (Carter and O'Morrow, 2006). When TRSs enter their first professional position, they are expected to formulate professional development (PD) plans for the future to ensure their ongoing acquisition of additional knowledge, experience, and skills in their field. This has become more important today than ever before because society and technology are changing and developing more rapidly, both in the United States and globally. For continually improving the safety and quality of care and services they provide clients, TRSs must always be learning new information; new skills; about new research in their field and related fields and its findings; new therapeutic and facilitative approaches, methods, techniques, and strategies; and new trends emerging in the health and human services field and the TR/RT discipline. Professional standards of practice therefore advise professional TRSs to design individual development plans and pursue continuing education. In fact, the NCTRC requires documenting continuing education units (CEUs)/PD points to keep the Certified Therapeutic Recreation Specialist (CTRS) credential once earned. TRSs take academic courses, participate in webinars, attend conferences, and conduct and publish research to earn these.

## CONTINUING EDUCATION
### HISTORICAL DEVELOPMENT

In the early days of the TR/RT profession, education in the 20th century concentrated on preparation. The first master's degree programs in recreation were offered at the University of West Virginia and University of Minnesota in 1951. Formal training in hospital recreation was offered by the University of Minnesota and University of North Carolina in the 1950s; six universities/colleges offered undergraduate/graduate hospital recreation programs by 1953. Professional development was advanced by conferences at the Universities of North Carolina and Minnesota in the 1950s and 1960s. Educational programs expanded dramatically in the 1970s, but then lost funding in the 1980s. Regardless, the Council on Higher Education Accreditation (CHEA, formerly Commission on Recognition of Postsecondary Accreditation) officially recognized the NRPA/AALR Accreditation Program in 1982, advancing acceptance of the TR/RT profession and discipline and of parks and recreation curricula. **Continuing education opportunities** increased as ATRA, its state affiliate chapters, the International Symposium on Therapeutic Recreation, and others sponsored conferences that provided professional development.

### DEVELOPMENTS IN THE LATE 20TH AND EARLY 21ST CENTURIES

Higher education institutions found challenges to TR/RT curriculum development during the late 1990s and early 2000s because of a gap between TRS educational preparation and accountability requirements. ATRA held a 1995 curriculum conference to address TR/RT education issues, producing a 1997 publication. Its 2008 revision, *Guidelines for Competency Assessment and Curriculum Planning for Recreational Therapy Practice* (West, Kinney, & Witman) updated curriculum guidelines, including emphasizing the need for safe, effective practices in healthcare settings where most TRSs work. To improve continuing education in TR/RT and facilitate TRS access to it, ATRA created the ATRA Academy, which developed webinars and audio programs. ATRA also published revised guidelines addressing inconsistencies in internship procedures and requirements in 1998. The former NTRS had published such guidelines in 1997. Both organizations advocated for and gained inclusion in the AMA's 1997–1998 *Health Professions Career and Education Directory*. Due to recommendations and inspiration from ATRA's curriculum conference, in 1997 the Council on Accreditation of Parks, Recreation, Tourism, and Related Professions (COAPRT) appointed a task force to review and recommend TR/RT accreditation standards and preparation competencies, including holistic health, inclusive practices, understanding caregiver roles, human service systems trends, and healthcare delivery models.

### EFFORTS TO INCREASE CONTINUING EDUCATION QUANTITY AND QUALITY

Experts in the field realized in the late 1990s that to satisfy both accountability measures and the needs of an increasingly diverse society with rapidly changing health and human service characteristics, TRS continuing education quantity and quality must increase. In 2000, The Alliance for Therapeutic Recreation established a work group for identifying issues and proposing strategies for addressing higher education's TR/RT curriculum challenges. Thereafter, a Joint Task Force on Higher Education created a strategic plan with goals of making professional TR/RT preparation programs stronger and more consistent. The Therapeutic Recreation Education Conference (TREC) convened in 2005 and 2009 to realize these goals. Its presentations are compiled in *Therapeutic Recreation Education: Challenges and Changes* (Carter & Folkerth, 2006). Concerns about entry-level preparation include multicultural competence and ethical education. The continuing education component of NCTRC's criteria requires CTRSs to earn CEUs through attending professional workshops, symposia, conferences, seminars; authoring professional publications; giving professional presentations; completing academic courses; internship supervision; and participating in official NCTRC test development, test item writing, and related activities, directly related to current NCTRC Job Analysis Knowledge Areas, to maintain certification/obtain recertification every five years.

## PROFESSIONAL ORGANIZATIONS

### NATIONAL THERAPEUTIC RECREATION SOCIETY (NTRS)

The National Therapeutic Recreation Society (NTRS) was a professional organization promoting the field of TR/RT and community recreation. The National Recreation and Park Association (NRPA) is an organization that includes the American Institute of Park Executives, National Recreation Association, National Conference on State Parks, American Association of Zoological Parks and Aquariums, the American Recreation Society, and its Hospital Recreation section. The National Association of Recreation Therapists, considering the potential benefits of affiliation with another recreation organization including 20,000 members, agreed to merge with NRPA in 1966, becoming its sixth branch renamed the National Therapeutic Recreation Society (NTRS). In addition to supporting NRPA goals, the NTRS identified purposes of collecting and disseminating TR/RT information; promoting participant rehabilitation via recreation; fostering a spirit of cooperation among all agencies and professions related to their cause; and developing facility, program, and personnel standards to improve services. However, organizational issues of governance, philosophical differences, autonomy needs, and controversy over developing an association definition and philosophical statement ultimately led to it forming a new organization in the 1980s and dissolving NTRS as a branch of NRPA in 2010.

### AMERICAN THERAPEUTIC RECREATION ASSOCIATION (ATRA)

The American Therapeutic Recreation Association (ATRA) was founded in 1984 in the District of Columbia as a nonprofit, incorporated grassroots organization to respond to increasing concerns regarding drastic changes in the healthcare industry. From its initial membership of 60 people, it grew to 2,200 members by 2014 with a goal of obtaining a membership of 10,000. It is the largest national membership organization to represent the needs, issues, and interests of the TR/RT profession. ATRA elects a board of directors including more than 35 volunteer committees and task forces, concentrating on various areas including evidence-based practice, diagnostic specialty groups, higher education, public policy, and health insurance coverage and reimbursement. Since its beginning, ATRA has placed emphasis on the importance of its membership's grassroots involvement. One way this is manifested is through its individual chapter affiliates. They give ATRA's board of directors continual information and feedback about issues confronting the TR/RT profession. Hence the board of directors has added a position of a chapter affiliate council chair, elected by the collective chapters. ATRA membership services include professional development, professional practice, advocacy, treatment networking, external affairs, educational services, competency guidelines, professional standards of practice, a code of ethics, annual and semi-annual conferences, and continuing education through ATRA Academy.

### ACTIVITIES AND COLLABORATIONS

The American Therapeutic Recreation Association (ATRA) advocated during the 1990s for including TR/RT services via participating in CARF International, the Joint Commission, and CMS; developing and distributing publications regarding reimbursement; and supporting legislative days on Capitol Hill and a paid lobbyist. It addressed healthcare reform issues through publications. ATRA collaborated with NTRS (1966–2010) in publishing protocol and reimbursement documents. Together they met with representatives of the federal Centers for Medicare and Medicaid Services (CMS) and the Joint Commission's Coalition of Rehabilitation Organizations about federal healthcare regulations and interpreting the TR/RT profession's position therein. ATRA and NTRS formed a Joint Task Force on Credentialing in 1996 to support state endeavors toward TR/RT recognition as healthcare providers in state regulations and codes. They established the Alliance for

Therapeutic Recreation in 1998, which formed a Joint Task Force on Long-Term Care in 1999 to support TRSs practicing in long-term care settings. The Alliance also addressed higher education/professional preparation issues in 2000 and 2001. "ATRA Day on the Hill", successful lobbying, legislative summits, and leadership training promoted TR/RT. ATRA accomplished great legislative impact in 2004 to include TR/RT in Medicare coverage in skilled nursing, inpatient rehabilitation, and inpatient psychiatric facilities.

## CONTINUING EDUCATION AND PROFESSIONAL GROWTH

Because the health and human services field is constantly changing, and professionals are continually publishing new research, TRSs must continually update and increase their knowledge and skills to maintain currency in their discipline and improve client services. NCTRC requires regular CTRS recertification, which requires continuing education. The American Therapeutic Recreation Association (ATRA), today's major TR/RT professional organization, offers many continuing education opportunities, including attending the ATRA annual conference, in 2015 held in Albuquerque, New Mexico. To help busy professionals earn CEUs and extend their knowledge, the ATRA Webinar Series enables online study. The website offers webinar replays and live calls to suit every participant's schedule. ATRA Annuals are collections of published research articles and post-tests, available for professionals to read for earning CEU credits up to five years after publication. Electronic versions are available to ATRA members. Membership includes subscription to the semi-monthly ATRA Newsletter, covering profession advances, industry news, and legislative alerts. Members can answer ten multiple-choice questions about newsletter content and submit their responses with $10 to earn 0.1 CEU. Reading archived editions also earns credit for up to one year. TR/RT professionals can also apply to have workshops certified by ATRA for CEU approval.

# ATRA CODE OF ETHICS

## INTRODUCTION

**ATRA's (1990) Code of Ethics** states that: TR provides treatment and recreation services to persons with disabilities or illnesses. The main purposes of treatment services are to remediate, rehabilitate, or restore to eliminate or decrease disability/disease impacts and improve functioning and independence. The main purposes of recreation services are to offer opportunities and resources for enhancing the wellbeing and health of clients. TR professionals are trained, registered, licensed, and/or certified to deliver TR/RT services. ATRA serves as an advocate for consumers and members of the TR/RT profession. The objectives of ATRA include furthering and supporting public awareness and understanding about TR/RT; developing and promoting professional TR/RT standards; advocating for the advancement of TR/RT services with medical treatment, educational services, habilitation services, and rehabilitation services for individuals who are in need of these services; conducting and supporting efforts in research and demonstration for the purpose of enhancing TR/RT service; and conducting and supporting educational opportunities for professionals who are studying and practicing in the discipline of TR/RT.

## PRINCIPLES

The ATRA Code of Ethics was most recently updated in 2009. It provides a structured guideline to ethical behavior of recreational therapists and is broken down into 10 guiding principles:

## PRINCIPLE 1: BENEFICENCE

Recreational Therapy personnel shall treat persons served in an ethical manner by actively making efforts to provide for their wellbeing by maximizing possible benefits and relieving, lessening, or minimizing possible harm.

## PRINCIPLE 2: NON-MALEFICENCE

Recreational Therapy personnel have an obligation to use their knowledge, skills, abilities, and judgment to help persons while respecting their decisions and protecting them from harm.

## PRINCIPLE 3: AUTONOMY

Recreational Therapy personnel have a duty to preserve and protect the right of each individual to make his or her own choices. Each individual is to be given the opportunity to determine his or her own course of action in accordance with a plan freely chosen. In the case of individuals who are unable to exercise autonomy with regard to their care, recreational therapy personnel have the duty to respect the decisions of their qualified legal representative.

## PRINCIPLE 4: JUSTICE

Recreational Therapy personnel are responsible for ensuring that individuals are served fairly and that there is equity in the distribution of services. Individuals should receive services without regard to race, color, creed, gender, sexual orientation, age, disease/disability, social and financial status.

## PRINCIPLE 5: FIDELITY

Recreational Therapy personnel have an obligation, first and foremost, to be loyal, faithful, and meet commitments made to persons receiving services. In addition, Recreational Therapy personnel have a secondary obligation to colleagues, agencies, and the profession.

## PRINCIPLE 6: VERACITY

Recreational Therapy personnel shall be truthful and honest. Deception, by being dishonest or omitting what is true, should always be avoided.

## PRINCIPLE 7: INFORMED CONSENT

Recreational Therapy personnel should provide services characterized by mutual respect and shared decision making. These personnel are responsible for providing each individual receiving service with information regarding the services, benefits, outcomes, length of treatment, expected activities, risk and limitations, including the professional's training and credentials. Informed consent is obtained when information needed to make a reasoned decision is provided by the professional to competent persons seeking services who then decide whether or not to accept the treatment.

## PRINCIPLE 8: CONFIDENTIALITY AND PRIVACY

Recreational Therapy personnel have a duty to disclose all relevant information to persons seeking services: they also have a corresponding duty not to disclose private information to third parties. If a situation arises that requires disclosure of confidential information about an individual the professional has the responsibility to inform the individual served of the circumstances.

## PRINCIPLE 9: COMPETENCE

Recreational Therapy personnel have the responsibility to maintain and improve their knowledge related to the profession and demonstrate current, competent practice to persons served. In addition, personnel have an obligation to maintain their credential.

## PRINCIPLE 10: COMPLIANCE WITH LAWS AND REGULATIONS

Recreational Therapy personnel are responsible for complying with local, state and federal laws, regulations and ATRA policies governing the profession of Recreational Therapy.

## Professional Behavior in the Context of the Code of Ethics

Many, if not all, principles of the American Therapeutic Recreation Association (ATRA)'s Code of Ethics relate to the **professional behavior** TRSs should demonstrate in their work. For example, Principles 1 and 2, Beneficence/Non-maleficence, require treating people ethically by both protecting them from harm and actively working toward their wellbeing. These are two aspects of professional behavior. Another is letting clients choose their treatment plans and actions freely, which Principle 3, Autonomy, requires. Professional TRSs must not discriminate in delivering services; Principle 4, Justice, stipulates this. Professional behavior also requires honesty and faithfulness to clients, co-workers, agencies, and the profession as Principle 5, Fidelity, states. Informing clients of their credentials and training; discussing limits, risks, durations, activities, results, and benefits of treatment; and obtaining informed consent, which Principles 6 and 7, Veracity/Informed Consent, are additional examples of professional behavior. TRSs must protect the privacy of clients' personal information, which Principle 8, Confidentiality and Privacy, addresses. Ongoing pursuit and documentation of additional expertise is another aspect of professional behavior, identified in Principle 9, Competence. Following legal requirements is also required for professional behavior, as affirmed in Principle 10, Compliance with Laws and Regulations.

## Characteristics and Features of Codes of Ethics in Health and Human Services

One feature that distinguishes professional practices in general from others is that professionals engage in **ethical behaviors**. Professions each develop their own codes of ethics. In the western world, these are traditionally based on Judeo-Christian principles for behavior that are considered morally responsible. These principles provide guidance to professionals for the actions they take in their work and provide expected standards of care by professionals to the public. While each profession has its own ethical code, those found in our society are very similar overall. For example, codes of ethical conduct for medical professionals subscribe to the Hippocratic Oath of first doing no harm and promoting wellbeing as well as preventing harm. Other health and human service professions have established similar codes. Another common feature of ethical codes in these fields is the principle of protecting patient/client information privacy and confidentiality. According to experts, ethical codes supply rules that emphasize the ideal in service, decrease competition within the discipline, and eliminate unqualified practitioners. In care/service fields, they also give social responsibility priority above financial remuneration and professional status. NTRS published a code of ethics; since its closing, ATRA offers a very similar ethical code.

## Regulatory Standards
### Joint Commission

The National Therapeutic Recreation Society (NTRS) had developed TR/RT standards for psychiatric facilities in 1971. The Joint Commission on Accreditation of Healthcare Organizations (JCAHO) developed its own standards based on those 1971 standards. A significant fact about the Joint Commission is that it was the first healthcare accrediting agency to adopt standards for therapeutic recreation. The Joint Commission is a nonprofit, independent organization. It grants certification and accreditation to more than 20,500 healthcare programs and organizations in the United States. Accreditation and certification by the Joint Commission is nationally acknowledged as a sign of an organization's quality and commitment to fulfilling high standards of performance. The Joint Commission's vision is that all Americans always receive health care in all settings that have the highest safety, quality, and value. The Joint Commission's mission is to improve health care for the public continually by collaborating with other stakeholders, evaluating healthcare organizations, and inspiring those organizations to excel at delivering safe, effective, valuable, high-quality care.

## COMMISSION ON ACCREDITATION AND REHABILITATION FACILITIES (CARF)

CARF (Commission on Accreditation of Rehabilitation Facilities), now known as CARF International, was founded in 1966, and today it includes CARF Europe, CARF Canada, and accreditation extending to South America, Asia, and Africa as well as the United States. Similar to the Joint Commission, CARF is a nonprofit, independent organization that serves as an external source of accreditation for health and human service providers, including providers of addiction and substance abuse treatment, behavioral health, children and youth services, business and service management networks, employment services, disability and medical rehabilitation, aging services, community services, home services, and providers of TR/RT services. CARF states that a provider's receiving its accreditation indicates that the provider is committed to serving its community, inviting feedback, and continuously improving its services. CARF focuses on improving the quality of services that providers deliver. It ensures that providers it accredits meet its high standards. CARF International accredits more than 64,000 services and programs and 8,000 service providers serving more than 8 million people annually in over 30,000 locations.

## CENTERS FOR MEDICARE AND MEDICAID SERVICES (CMS)

CMS stands for the Centers for Medicare and Medicaid Services, a federal agency. Formerly the Health Care Financing Administration (HCFA), it was renamed in 2001. A 1965 amendment to the 1935 Social Security Act incorporated the Medicare program. Medicare Part A provides hospital insurance, Part B medical insurance. Funded by employer and employee contributions, Medicare covers hospitalization, outpatient hospital, physician, skilled nursing, home health, and hospice care to people aged 65+/with specified disabilities, but does not cover long-term nursing home custodial care. Federally funded prescription medication insurance became available, effective 2006, via the Medicare Prescription Drug Improvement and Modernization Act, passed in 2003. Medicaid is also a federal assistance program, but administered by individual states. It covers most medical needs for people of all ages who are eligible for Medicaid. It does not cover long-term care in assisted living facilities, but does cover long-term care in nursing homes, adult care homes, hospital care, physician services, medications, supplies, and caregiver income-expense gaps. CMS's 1987 Omnibus Budget Reconciliation Act (OBRA), effective 1990, requires state assessment and reporting of long-term facility resident outcomes receiving Medicare/Medicaid, including documentation of physician-ordered RT/TR active treatment outcomes and activity preferences.

## OLDER AMERICAN ACT

Congress passed the Older Americans Act (OAA) in 1965 among President Lyndon Johnson's Great Society reforms, addressing concerns about inadequate community social services for senior citizens, reauthorized 2006–2011. Funding has not met inflation since. 2014 reauthorization for 2014–2018 appropriations, not enacted, was referred to committee. While many other federal programs provide aging services, OAA is the primary mechanism, authorizing state grants for aging-related personnel training, research and development, social services, community planning, and establishing the Administration on Aging (AoA) via Title II. Title III allocated federal funds for, and mandated creating, 56 state aging agencies. Title IV created projects, including for civic engagement, computer training, rural area healthcare services, and Native American programs. Title V created a program to engage low-income senior citizens in volunteer and community service opportunities. Title VI created grants for programs focusing on Native American aging. Title VII established state grants for programs to protect vulnerable elder rights. Amendments established the National Family Caregiver support program for information, training, counseling, and respite care; funded state elder abuse detection; required comprehensive home and community long-term care/aging-in-place service systems. OAA authorizes almost 20,000 service providers and funds 629 area agencies and Aging and Disability Resource Centers.

The Older Americans Act (OAA), originally passed in 1965 and amended numerous times since, established the Administration on Aging (AoA). This administration is in charge of the oversight of various programs for aging adults, including local Area Agency on Aging (AAA) services, day care centers, low-cost transportation services, and nutrition centers. Amendments include establishing the National Family Caregiver Support Program, providing families/other caregivers of disabled, ill, and frail older adults with respite care, counseling, information, and training; grants to US states for identifying elder abuse and funding for Aging and Disability Resource Centers (ADRCs) for providing older adults with disabilities assistance to access information and options for long-term care; and the requirement that the AoA and local AAAs plan comprehensive community-based and home-based service systems to enable older people with long-term care needs to "age in place" (at home). TRSs can find information and resources on funding, transportation, medication, and legislation regarding aging adults from local AAAs; public Park and Recreation Departments' senior centers; at the National Institutes of Health (NIH), National Institute on Aging (NIA), and Centers for Medicare and Medicaid Services (CMS) websites, among others.

## REHABILITATION ACT

The Rehabilitation Act of 1973 requires all federal employers and programs and activities receiving federal funding to provide equal access to persons with disabilities.

- This law's **Section 502** also established the Access Board (the Architectural and Transportation Barriers Compliance Board) to enforce compliance with the Architectural Barriers Act (ABA), to ensure that design standards were developed to enable compliance and to further equal access throughout society.
- **Section 508** of the Rehabilitation Act was amended in 1998 to increase the requirements for federal employers and federally funded agencies/programs to provide equal access to any electronic and information technology they develop, obtain, maintain, or utilize for people with disabilities. Federal employees and members of the public with disabilities must have equal access to computers, software, peripheral devices, electronic office equipment, etc., unless this constitutes an "undue burden." National security systems are exempt.
- **Section 510,** enacted in 2010, extends and reforms health care provision to include independent access to and use of medical diagnostic equipment in hospitals, emergency rooms, medical clinics, physicians' offices, and other medical settings by persons with disabilities to the fullest extent possible.

## SECTION 504

Under the US Rehabilitation Act of 1973, Section 504 protects people with disabilities against discrimination based on their disabilities by any employers and organizations receiving financial assistance from any federal agency/department, including the Department of Health and Human Services (DHHS). Many hospitals, nursing homes, mental health centers, and human services programs are included among these employers and organizations. Individuals with disabilities may not be excluded or denied equal opportunities to receive services and benefits from federally funded programs. Section 504 defines the rights of individuals with disabilities for access to and participation in program services and benefits. Disabilities are defined as physical or mental impairments limiting one or more major life activities substantially. This includes people with a history of such impairments, even if in remission, if they would significantly limit a major life activity if they became active again. Breathing, walking, seeing, hearing, speaking, learning, doing manual tasks, working, and self-care are included among major life activities. AIDS, alcoholism, blindness/visual impairments, cancer, deafness/hearing loss, diabetes, drug addiction, heart disease, and mental illness are examples of substantially limiting impairments, even with help from medications/aids/devices.

## ARCHITECTURAL BARRIERS ACT

The Architectural Barriers Act (ABA) of 1968 was enacted "to ensure that certain buildings financed with federal funds are so designed and constructed as to be accessible to the physically handicapped." Under the Rehabilitation Act of 1973, Section 502 established the Architectural and Transportation Barriers Compliance Board, later called the Access Board. This board was created to enforce compliance with the ABA after Congress determined that the compliance of state and local agencies receiving federal funding was irregular and that there were no initiatives in process for establishing federal design standards for accessibility. The board was additionally charged with the duties of proposing solutions to the problems addressed in the ABA concerning environmental barriers; developing and maintaining guidelines as the bases for the standards issued under the ABA; and promoting access to public facilities, buildings, and programs receiving federal funding throughout all areas of American society. According to the law, this board's functions also include providing "appropriate technical assistance" and "advisory information" to individual persons, groups, or entities who have duties or rights addressed by Titles II and III of the Americans with Disabilities Act (ADA) of 1990 "with respect to overcoming architectural, transportation, and communication barriers."

## OMNIBUS BUDGET RECONCILIATION ACT

The Omnibus Budget Reconciliation Act (OBRA), passed 1987, effective 1990, requires states to evaluate and document outcomes for Medicare and Medicaid recipients residing in long-term care facilities to the federal government's Centers for Medicare and Medicaid Services (CMS). The Minimum Data Set (MDS 3.0) is a tool for assessment, reimbursement, and quality improvement that OBRA requires long-term care facilities to use to evaluate each resident. Section F, Preferences for Customary Routine and Activities, and Section O, Special Treatments and Procedures, of the MDS require TRSs to document each resident's activity preferences and the resident's outcomes that are attributed to the effects of TR/RT services. The data that TRSs report under these OBRA regulations are used by the government for calculating the case mix rates of the reimbursements that it pays directly to the service providers. Hence these reporting requirements have a direct impact on whether and how much TRSs are paid for the services they provide to clients who are insured by Medicare and Medicaid.

## AMERICANS WITH DISABILITIES ACT

The Americans with Disabilities Act (ADA) was signed by President George H. W. Bush in 1990. This law was modeled on the 1964 Civil Rights Act, which prohibits discrimination against people on the basis of race, color, religion, sex, or national origin, extending the same civil rights protections to persons with disabilities; and also on Section 504 of the 1973 Rehabilitation Act, which requires federal employment, and programs and activities receiving funding from federal agencies, to provide access to people with disabilities. Similarly, the ADA asserts the rights of people with disabilities to equal opportunity in employment and access to public facilities, buildings, programs, and activities, including leisure and recreational facilities, programs, and activities. The Disability Rights section of the US Department of Justice (DOJ) is responsible for protecting rights of people with disabilities relative to the ADA. DOJ regulations for implementing the ADA in state and local governments are in ADA Title II, and in businesses and nonprofit service providers in Title III. ADA Titles II and III also contain enforceable standards for accessible facility and building design, construction, alteration, barrier removal, and building and program accessibility.

## INCLUSION OF LEISURE AND RECREATION EXPERIENCES AMONG PUBLIC ENTITIES

The ADA prohibits discrimination against any individual "on the basis of disability" from "full and equal enjoyment of ... goods, services, facilities, privileges, advantages, or accommodations of any place of public accommodation by any person who owns, leases (or leases to), or operates a place of public accommodation." This includes "denial of participation" (denying individuals or groups the opportunity to benefit from or participate in those things based on disability); "participation in unequal benefit" (giving individuals or groups with disabilities opportunities not equal to those given to others to benefit or participate in); and "separate benefit" (giving them goods, services, facilities, privileges, advantages, or accommodations different or separate from those given others, unless this is necessary to give them equally effective opportunities as others are given). It also requires "integrated settings" (offering the aforementioned things "in the most integrated setting appropriate to the needs of the individual"); "opportunity to participate" (they must not deny people with disabilities a chance to participate in non-separate programs and activities regardless of the existence of separate programs and activities).

## REGULATIONS DEFINING STANDARDS OF PUBLIC FACILITY ACCESS

The Americans with Disabilities Act (ADA) includes Accessibility Guidelines (ADAAG) defining how public facilities and areas should be accessible to people with disabilities. The American National Standards Institute (ANSI) publishes standards of physical accessibility for public facilities. The Uniform Federal Accessibility Standards (UFAS) is another source of such standards. These publications define the criteria by which outdoor areas, parking lots, building entrances, ramps, restrooms, stairs, telephones, water fountains, showers, swimming pools, and other elements of public facilities must be designed to allow access by all adults and children, including those with various disabilities. The ADAAG standards include supplements defining accessibility criteria for recreation facilities, outdoor environments, and play areas. Standards require play areas to contain a minimum number of play components, at ground level and elevated, plus transfer systems, ramps, and accessible surfaces and routes. Exercise machines and equipment; bowling lanes; swimming pools, wading pools, spas; golf and miniature golf courses; fishing platforms and piers; boating facilities; amusement rides; and firing ranges/facilities are included in recreation facilities. Outdoor environments include picnic and camping grounds, beaches, and trails.

## *INDIVIDUALS WITH DISABILITIES EDUCATION ACT*

The Individuals with Disabilities Education Act (IDEA) guarantees students with disabilities the right to a free, appropriate public education (FAPE) in the least restrictive environment (LRE) possible for the individual. It guarantees each student the right to have an individualized education program (IEP) developed for him or her by a multidisciplinary educational team, specifying which special education and related services the student requires to benefit from and succeed in public education, the student's educational goals and objectives, and a schedule for meeting and ways for measuring these. The IEP team can include the student, parents, advocates, classroom teachers, special education teachers, educational specialists, therapists, and others involved. The law specifies that student IEPs include transition plans started at age 14. Parents have rights, called Procedural Safeguards under **Subpart E,** to: have these rights available; FAPE for their child; confidentiality; inspect and review their child's educational records; participate in identification/evaluation/placement meetings; receive prior written notice of these; give/deny consent to school actions, and disagree with school decisions, regarding their child; determination appeals; and dispute resolution due process. **Part B** addresses educating children aged 3–22 years with disabilities; **Part C,** added later, addresses educating babies and toddlers aged 0–3 years with disabilities.

## STANDARDS OF PRACTICE

The National Therapeutic Recreation Society (NTRS) developed **standards of practice** for TR/RT in psychiatric facilities in 1971, providing the foundation for the Joint Commission standards. The Joint Commission was the first healthcare accrediting agency to adopt TR/RT standards. Also in 1971, with a US Department of Health, Education and Welfare-funded grant, Doris Berryman developed recreation standards for residential institutions, which then became the model for two documents: *Standards for the Practice of Therapeutic Recreation Service* and *Guidelines for the Administration of Therapeutic Recreation Service in Clinical and Residential Facilities*, published by NTRS in 1980. Previously another document, *Guidelines for Community-Based Recreation Programs for Special Populations,* published in 1979, contained similar standards of practice for community TR/RT services. To assure quality control of proliferating TR/RT academic preparation curricula, the National Recreation and Park Association (NRPA) and American Association of Physical Activity and Recreation (AAPAR, then American Association for Leisure and Recreation/AALR) developed a process to review and accredit university/college parks and recreation curricula, the Council on Accreditation of Parks, Recreation, Tourism, and Related Professions (COAPRT), including the first undergraduate and graduate-level TR/RT specialization accreditation.

### DEVELOPMENT

The National Therapeutic Recreation Society (NTRS), a former professional organization under the National Recreation and Park Association (NRPA) until 2010, developed standards of practice for the TR/RT profession. The American Therapeutic Recreation Association (ATRA) is a current professional organization that has also published standards of practice. ATRA has addressed healthcare reform issues related to practice standards in its publication, *Recreational Therapy: A Summary of Health Outcomes* (1994). Subsequently, NTRS and ATRA collaborated on a joint initiative regarding how the TR/RT profession could respond to healthcare reform, and published a joint statement, *Therapeutic Recreation: Responding to the Challenges of Healthcare Reform.* These two organizations also published protocol and reimbursement documents and interacted with the Joint Commission, the Commission on Accreditation of Rehabilitation Facilities (CARF) International, and the Centers for Medicare and Medicaid Services (CMS) to interpret the position of the TR/RT profession with respect to federal regulations on health care. The ATRA most recently published the ATRA Standards of Practice of Recreational Therapy and Self-Assessment Guide in 2013 that was then revised in 2015. Professional organizations have continued to create and revise TR/RT practice standards.

### PRACTICE LEVELS DEFINED BY NCTRC STANDARDS

Between 1981 and 1992, the National Council for Therapeutic Recreation Certification (NCTRC) defined Professional and Assistant levels of practice. In 1993, the National Commission for Certifying Agencies (NCCA) accredited NCTRC and received federal trademark registration of its Certified Therapeutic Recreation Specialist (CTRS) credential. After identifying an insufficient number of applicants for Assistant-level certification, NCTRC discontinued this level in 1999. To become a CTRS, an applicant must complete a bachelor's or higher degree with credit hours specified in coursework defined by the Professional Knowledge Domains, successfully pass a computer mastery test, and complete an internship supervised by a CTRS for a specified number of hours, performing tasks defined by the Job Task Domains. The CTRS indicates that the holder practices with no intent to cause clients any harm and according to "most current therapeutic professional standards and ethical guidelines." The Specialty Certification Program for qualified CTRSs includes Developmental Disabilities, Geriatrics, Physical Medicine/Rehabilitation, Community Inclusion, and Behavioral Health services. This certification recognizes advanced practice competencies in CTRSs.

## RECENT UPDATES TO STANDARDS OF PRACTICE

The American Therapeutic Recreation Association (ATRA) updated its standards of practice in 1990, 1993, 1998, 2000, 2001, 2009, 2013, and 2015. The National Therapeutic Recreation Society (NTRS, closed 2010) updated its practice standards in 1990, 1994, 1995, 1998, 2001, and 2003. The 1995, 1998, and 2003 revisions included TR process implementation assessment criteria and paraprofessional standards. Such revisions are necessary for making the TR/RT field a valid learned-service profession. Being self-regulated, these standards are regarded as proof that the profession is maturing. As a result, the TR/RT profession's having criteria in place for governing its practice contributes to the perception that it is more closely approaching acknowledgement as a real profession. The application of standards of practice for defining the scope of TR/RT services and measuring the quality of service delivery is another index of the profession's growing maturity. Among changes and additions to ATRA standards of practice in 1993, 1998, and 2000 was the addition of a self-assessment instrument for professional and paraprofessional-level practitioners' implementation of programming and administrative practices. Thorough field research at clinical agencies nationwide affirmed the suitability of ATRA's document as a professional accountability instrument.

## ATRA STANDARDS OF PRACTICE

The American Therapeutic Recreation Association (ATRA) Standards of Practice include 12 standards in addition to a Self-Assessment Guide to help recreational therapists maintain quality of care:

- standard 1 covers assessment.
- Standard 2 covers treatment planning.
- Standard 3 involves plan implementation.
- Standard 4 pertains to reassessment and evaluation.
- Standard 5 addresses discharge and transition planning.
- Standard 6 covers prevention, safety planning, and risk management.
- Standard 7 addresses ethical conduct.
- standard 8 describes how to make a written plan of operation.
- Standard 9 identifies criteria for staff qualifications and competency assessment.
- Standard 10 addresses the subject of quality management.
- Standard 11 covers the topic of resource management.
- Standard 12 provides guidelines for program evaluation and research.

An additional section in the ATRA Standards of Practice is the Self-Assessment Guide. This includes a Scoring Summary Worksheet; a Documentation Audit; a Management Audit; an Outcome Assessment; a Competency Assessment; and a Clinical Performance Appraisal to assist TRSs in conducting self-assessments of their own competencies and performance according to the standards.

## NCB AND NRPA CERTIFICATIONS

Job analyses made by the National Certification Board (NCB) in 1999 and 2006 led to the merging of TR/RT test specifications into three main content areas: programming, management, and operations. The NCB's job analyses also reinforced the importance of parks and recreation professionals' engaging in inclusive practices. The former Certified Leisure Professional (CLP) credential was renamed in early 2000 as Certified Park and Recreation Professional (CPRP). The first computerized CPRP examination, like the first computerized CTRS examination, was administered in 2001. As with the elimination of the Assistant level of the CTRS credential owing to an insufficient number of candidates, the CPRP credential was also revised to only a Professional level. Strategic planning identified goals of administering a national-level plan, instead of having respective states each administer a national plan, and establishing a Mastery level. In 2010 the National Recreation and Park Association (NRPA), consulting with the NCB, undertook a job task analysis for potentially implementing executive-/manager-level certification. NCB and the National Commission for Therapeutic Recreation Certification (NCTRC) agreed jointly in 2009 to begin designing specialty certifications. State-level CPRP plans were transitioned to national-level NRPA management from 2008–2010. Specialization areas as of 2022 include adaptive sports and recreation, behavioral health, community inclusion services, developmental disabilities, geriatrics, pediatrics, and physical medicine/rehabilitation. Specialization certification lasts for five years after which point the certification must be renewed.

# Assessment

## Conduct Assessment Process

### THERAPEUTIC RELATIONSHIP

#### LEVELS OF COMMUNICATION

Five levels of communication that inform personal interaction:

| Level | Goal | Description |
|-------|------|-------------|
| 5 | Cliché conversation | standard everyday greetings. These enable people to acknowledge one another in social contexts without inviting additional involvement. For example, it is inappropriate to respond to "How are you?" by describing one's medical conditions in detail. |
| 4 | Reporting facts | People share general information about impersonal topics (e.g., weather, sports, fashion, reading, entertainment, etc.). |
| 3 | Personal ideas and judgments | People express some personal information (e.g., opinions, ideas, decisions). They react to listener feedback: if the listener seems interested, they may share more; if the listener seems bored, confused, or judgmental, they will likely withhold additional sharing. |
| 2 | Feelings and emotions | People will only share at this level when mutual trust and sharing have developed. Expressing deeply seated emotions is reserved for close friendships and intimate relationships between people who genuinely care about each other. |
| 1 | Peak communication | This rare, deepest level of interaction involves near-perfect, reciprocal understanding, total honesty and openness in a relationship of all-embracing intimacy. Some people never, and many people seldom, experience this. |

#### INTERPERSONAL FACILITATION SKILLS

In therapeutic/helping relationships, practitioners can overcome client intimidation at environment, circumstances, and/or professional presence by establishing relaxed, open atmospheres. One facilitating technique is *leading/inviting requests* (anticipating client needs and encouraging clients to make requests or ask questions). Another is *responding/informing* clients by giving them factual, objective information at levels consistent with their understanding. When responding to questions/requests, therapists must *interpret* them properly. For example, a patient's question about why hospital personnel are repeatedly drawing blood would be interpreted differently according to age: an adult's underlying fear could be that doctors suspect a more serious medical problem; a child's underlying fear could be that he or she will run out of blood and die from repeated drawings. Responding also includes appropriate action. Therapists convey *warmth* and caring through eye contact, appropriate touch, vocal tone, eye/facial expression, openness to both positive and negative expressions, and respecting silence. *Attending* skills include appropriate social distance; culturally appropriate eye contact, without intimidating staring or a frequently averted gaze signaling unease; open, relaxed posture; equal body orientation (e.g., seated with clients in wheelchairs); avoiding interfering gestures while clients communicate; not interrupting/redirecting client messages. Active, reflective *listening* is another important facilitation skill.

## PROVIDING LEADERSHIP TO CLIENTS

TRSs must always be professional. To help clients effectively, they must engender trust. This requires protecting the confidentiality of client information and not sharing it with friends or family. TRSs should protect not only clients' information confidentiality, but also their humanity and dignity. They must consider clients in relationship to their environments. Families, social networks, and agencies and their interactions with clients can afford both assets to and detractions from client autonomy, competence, and growth. Professionalism also requires objectivity, which is compromised by becoming overinvolved with clients. However, TRSs should partner/collaborate with clients. Utilizing clients' own resources engages their active participation in the processes of change and growth and empowers them to take responsibility for their own wellbeing. While maintaining professionalism, TRSs should still be themselves, seeking colleagues' support for authentic behavior and sharing fears/anxieties with them. They should consider the multicultural elements of the APIE process, including the impacts of culture on both client and therapist roles and beliefs about health and illness. They should reflect their consideration of these impacts in culturally sensitive practices.

## RECOMMENDED INTERVENTIONS

To foster secure, safe environments for growth toward independence and personal fulfillment, TRSs should provide as much structure as is required. Clients with psychological disorders need stronger structure. To increase socialization, sequence activities with progressive levels of interaction. Severely disturbed clients may start participating in parallel/1:1 interactions; progress to structured, individualized/small-group activities; and eventually transition to direct social interactions in larger group activities. Touch, albeit highly useful for furthering interpersonal relationships, is potentially problematic: some clients are frightened or offended by it; teens/young adults can interpret hugs differently than children do; needy individuals can misconstrue their import. Therefore, use discretion with physical contact. Planning widely varied activities addresses all clients' cultural and personal interests and needs. Consider each client's uniqueness. For clients with limited interests, offer new activities, affording growth opportunities. Although medication reactions and other circumstances can restrict activity, encourage clients' active participating, not passive observing/spectating. Increase involvement by including every client in some aspect (e.g., judging, officiating, scorekeeping) of activities. Communicate genuine interest in client wellbeing through persistence, firmness, and consistency. Balance enthusiasm with sensitivity to current client status. Motivate through strong helping relationships and example/modeling.

## PROFESSIONAL BOUNDARIES

The RT must maintain **professional boundaries** and remember that a client is not the same as a family member or friend despite long-term relationships (in some cases) and should avoid sharing inappropriate personal information (such as telephone number, personal life details, or personal problems) or giving advice unrelated to treatment (such as about client's family problems). The RT should avoid all inappropriate touching or relationships and should avoid discussion of or contact with clients on social media. The RT should avoid accepting or giving gifts as this may result in an unanticipated sense of obligation or expectation. As acts of kindness, RTs, especially with in-home care, often give clients extra attention and may offer to do favors, such as cooking or shopping, and may become overly invested in the clients' lives. While this may benefit clients in the short term, it can establish a relationship of increasing dependency and obligation that does not resolve the ongoing needs of clients or family and may make the RT liable for civil or legal action if behavior is misunderstood.

## HUMAN GROWTH AND DEVELOPMENT
### PHYSICAL GROWTH AND DEVELOPMENT FROM BIRTH THROUGH EARLY ADULTHOOD

Before **birth and during infancy**, human growth follows two patterns. Cephalocaudal (head-to-tail) growth begins at the top, proceeding downward. Proximodistal (near-to-far) growth begins in the center, proceeding outward. Birth weight doubles within five months. Weight almost triples in a year; height grows 1½ times birth length. By 2 years, children gain ¼–½ lb monthly, reaching around 1/5 adult weight and almost half adult height. In **early childhood**, average growth is 5–7 lb, 2½ inches yearly. Children lose "baby fat." Head-to-body proportion becomes less oversized. Female-male size differences are minor. Middle and late childhood involve slow, steady growth, around 2–3 inches and 5–7 lb yearly. Muscle mass and tone increase, body fat decreases; strength doubles. During **adolescence**, puberty involves rapid physical and sexual maturation. Both sexes gain height and weight; females' growth spurts and pubertal changes begin two years before males'. **Young adults** usually attain peak physical performance between 19–26 years, but fatty tissue begins increasing in the mid-to-late 20s; muscle strength and tone start declining by age 30. The eyes' lenses begin losing elasticity, causing difficulty focusing and farsightedness; hearing starts declining near the end of **early adulthood**.

### MOTOR DEVELOPMENT IN INFANCY AND CHILDHOOD

Babies are born with built-in **motor reactions** to stimuli, called reflexes. These include blinking, rooting, sucking, grasping; tonic neck, stepping, and swimming reflexes; and the Moro/startle and Babinski reflexes. Blinking is permanent; the others all disappear at ages ranging from 2–12 months. Gross motor skills involve large-muscle functions like posture, arm movements, and walking. Fine motor skills involve small-muscle functions like using hands and fingers to manipulate small objects. Babies lift heads while prone within 1 month; raise chests supported by arms within 2–4 months; roll over around 2–5 months; support some weight on legs by 3–6+ months; sit unsupported around 4–7 months; stand, supported, between 5–10 months; pull up between 6–10 months; "cruise" using furniture from 7–12 months; stand easily, unsupported, between 10–14 months; and easily walk independently between 11–14+ months. Toddlers can climb steps by 13–18 months; walk fast/run short distances stiffly, walk backward, throw and kick balls, jump in place, and balance squatting by 18–24 months. Preschoolers develop automaticity in gross motor skills; by age 4, fine motor coordination gains significant precision. Middle childhood brings greater ease, independence, and precision for writing, etc. By 10–12 years, children develop manipulative skills similar to adults'.

### PHYSICAL CHANGES THAT OCCUR DURING MIDDLE AND LATE ADULTHOOD

In **mid-adulthood**, lost collagen and fat make skin sag and wrinkle. Hair grays and thins. Fingernails and toenails develop ridges, brittleness, and thickening. Teeth yellow. Due to vertebral bone loss and shrinking cartilage, most male adults lose ½" in height from age 30–50, another ¾" from 50–70. Females may lose up to 2" from age 25–75. Body fat doubles from adolescence to middle adulthood, from 10%–20%. Muscle strength and mass decrease around 1%–2% annually after age 50. Joint function declines, causing stiffness and more difficult movement. Bone density decreases progressively, accelerating in the 50s; women lose bone about twice as rapidly as men. Bones fracture more readily, with slower healing. Near vision and focus decline most from ages 40–59. Hearing declines, initially for high frequencies. High blood pressure and cholesterol become more common. Deep sleep decreases, wakefulness increases. Some individuals develop diseases/health problems in middle adulthood; generally accidents, colds, and allergy symptoms become less frequent. Women undergo menopause, men smaller hormonal decreases. **Older adults** lose height and typically weight. Movement slows. Visual acuity, depth perception, color vision, hearing acuity and discrimination decline—more after age 75 than from 65–74. Lung capacity decreases 40% from age 20–80.

## THEORIES OF HUMAN DEVELOPMENT
### PIAGET'S STAGES OF COGNITIVE DEVELOPMENT

Piaget termed infancy and early childhood the *sensorimotor* stage, when babies/children learn by responding to *sensory* input from environmental stimuli with *motor* reactions. By interacting with the environment, they learn how it functions and ways to affect it. Piaget called toddlerhood the *preoperational* stage: children think intuitively and cannot perform mental operations or follow logical sequences. They are *egocentric*, unable to see others' physical or mental perspectives; have *animistic* thinking, attributing human qualities to inanimate objects; and *magical thinking*, believing their thoughts/words/actions cause external events. They *"centrate"* on one object property, not understanding liquid is the same amount in a tall, thin or short, wide container; clay is the same amount shaped in a round ball or a long, thin rope; toys are the same number clustered together or spread apart. They believe several pieces of a cookie equal more than one whole cookie. Piaget described middle childhood as the *concrete operations* stage: children can think logically about concrete objects/events they can see/touch/manipulate. They *"decentrate"*—can now conserve quantities despite shape or arrangement—and *reverse* operations. Preadolescents/adolescents enter what Piaget termed *formal operations*: they can perform mental operations without concrete objects/events and understand abstract concepts like justice and ethics.

### FREUD'S THEORY OF PSYCHOSEXUAL DEVELOPMENT

Freud felt the personality was formed by adolescence, so his theory did not encompass the entire lifespan. He believed procreation and death were the basic instincts driving human life. Freud proposed three basic personality structures:

- The *id* generates impulses.
- The *ego* governs realistic self-preservation.
- The *superego* provides a conscience.

He defined a number of defense mechanisms produced by the ego to protect the self from threats. Freud's stage theory of development emphasized erogenous zones as focal points where pleasure is derived in each age range. Infants are in the *oral* stage, centered on nursing; sustenance is a main issue. Toddlers are in the *anal* stage, centered on toilet-training; control is an issue. Young children enter the *phallic* stage, centered on discovering the genitals; exploration is an issue. Middle/school-age children are in the *latency* stage, deferring genital interests for new academic and social activities; learning and socialization are important. Adolescents enter the *genital* stage as puberty reawakens sexual urges; sexuality and intimacy become more important.

## ERIKSON'S THEORY OF PSYCHOSOCIAL DEVELOPMENT

Erikson's first five stages of psychosocial development were influenced by Freud's; however, his theory encompasses the lifespan and emphasizes psychosocial over psychosexual development. Each stage centers on resolving a nuclear conflict with positive/negative outcomes.

- **Trust vs. Mistrust** (0-1.5 years): The infant develops trust in those who provide basic care and safety. Success leads to the virtue of hope.
- **Autonomy vs. Shame and Doubt** (1.5-3 years): Tasks are performed independently and there should be freedom to test independence. Success leads to confidence.
- **Initiative vs. Guilt** (3-5 years): More independence and initiative in decision-making develops. Success leads to security in actions.
- **Industry vs. Inferiority** (5-12 years): The peer group plays a larger role in self-esteem. There is confidence in achieving goals. Success leads to feeling competent.
- **Identity vs. Role Confusion** (12-18 years): The child is searching for self-identity and exploring who they want to be as an adult. Success leads to a positive self-esteem.
- **Intimacy vs. Isolation** (18-40 years): Committed relationships are formed. Success leads to security within a relationship.
- **Generativity vs. Stagnation** (40-65 years): Careers are established and there is giving back to society. Success leads to feelings of productivity.
- **Ego integrity vs. Despair** (65+ years): There is reflection on whether their active years have been productive. Success leads to not feeling guilty or unsuccessful with their life's work.

## SELF-DETERMINATION THEORY

The Self-Determination Theory (SDT) (Ryan and Deci) suggests that human behavior seeks to meet three primary needs—competence, autonomy, and relatedness—necessary for growth and development. SDT focuses on how motivation factors into these needs:

- **Intrinsic motivation**: Individuals seek challenges and explore, but inherent motivation requires nurturing. To sustain intrinsic motivation, the individual must retain autonomy and demonstrate competence. Intrinsic motivation is diminished by both a system of external rewards (which places the focus outside of the individual) and negative pressures, such as threats or punishments.
- **Extrinsic motivation**: Individual act in order to obtain an external outcome, such as a reward or respect. Extrinsic motivation that the individual endorses (exercising in order to feel better) is more successful than that for which the individual feels little value.

Six elements that are part of SDT include: Cognitive evaluation (inherent motivation without concern for rewards), organismic integration (the continuum of extrinsic motivation), causality orientations (different orientations—autonomy, control, and amotivation), basic psychological needs (autonomy, competence, and relatedness necessary for psychological wellbeing), goal contents (distinguishes intrinsic and extrinsic goals), and relatedness (ties with friends, partners).

## EXPERIENTIAL LEARNING THEORY

The Experiential Learning Theory (Kolb) suggests that learning occurs through four stages of experience: concrete experience (actively carrying out an activity or experience), reflective observation (thinking about the activity or experience), abstract conceptualization (trying to conceptualize a model), and active experimentation (testing the model). While progressing through all stages is a necessary component of learning, some people prefer a particular style of learning:

- **Accommodative**: Prefers to learn through a combination of concrete experience and active experimentation, solves problems through trial and error, and tends to complete tasks.
- **Assimilative**: Prefers abstract concepts and reflective observation and is more interested in abstract ideas than people and applying ideas.
- **Divergent**: Prefers concrete experience and reflective observations and is imaginative with good ideas and is emotional. Likes working with people.
- **Convergent**: Prefers abstract concepts and active experimentation and prefers dealing with things to people.

## HUMANISTIC THEORIES OF HUMAN BEHAVIOR

Humanistic theories evolved from the human potential movement. Two of the most famous are Maslow's and Rogers' theories.

- **Maslow** proposed a hierarchy of needs, visualized in pyramid form. At base are physiological needs: sleep, water, food, and being warm; then needs for safety and security. Psychological needs follow: for love, friendship, and belonging; then esteem needs for feelings of accomplishment and prestige. Above these are self-actualization needs to fulfill one's highest potential, including creatively. Maslow proposed more basic needs must be met before each successive level could be fulfilled.

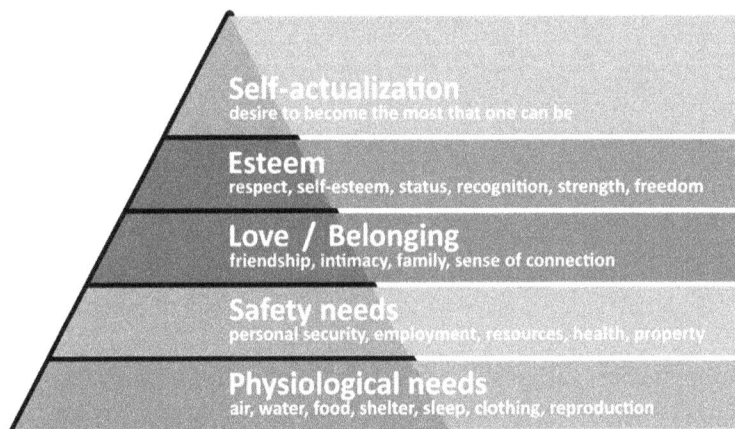

- **Carl Rogers** developed a person-centered humanistic theory. Self/self-concept was central to Rogers' theory. He agreed with Maslow about the human need for self-actualization, finding this requires environments offering open, genuine self-disclosure; acceptance (unconditional positive regard); and empathy (being listened to and understood). Rogers said one's self-image/actual behavior must be congruent with one's ideal self for self-actualization. He distinguished between unconditional positive regard, when parents love a child for who/what he or she is, and conditional positive regard, when parents only love/approve of a child on condition of certain behaviors. He identified people constantly seeking/depending on others' approval as having experienced conditional positive regard in childhood.

## ALBERT BANDURA'S SOCIAL LEARNING THEORY

Albert Bandura countered the theories of behaviorists who believed direct personal interactions with environmental stimuli were required in order to change people's behavior. He found people

43

could observe others interacting with environmental stimuli; be motivated to receive reinforcements as others did for their behaviors; remember the observed behaviors; and then imitate them, thus learning new behaviors. In response to questions whether media content that children watched could influence their actions, Bandura conducted landmark experiments exposing young children to videos featuring violence. Bandura and his associates observed the children's aggressive behaviors increased after viewing these videos. Thus, he proved children who watch violent content on TV and in movies are influenced to behave more aggressively/violently. This finding supported the concern of parents and educators about children's exposure to violent content and refuted the denials of others that children's behavior was not affected by media content they experienced. Knowing that young children cannot distinguish fiction or fantasy from reality adds weight to Bandura's proof of vicarious/observational learning to inform caution about children's media exposure.

## CONDITIONS FOR OBSERVATIONAL LEARNING

Bandura emphasized the social context in which learning occurs and the major roles of observation and motivation in learning. Bandura also proposed environmental, behavioral, and personal factors influence each other mutually/reciprocally (reciprocal determinism). He found people function via continual interactions among contextual, cognitive, and behavioral influences; students learn through reinforcements they/ their classmates receive, self-beliefs and thoughts, and interpreting classroom contexts. Contrary to behaviorism's environmental determinism, Bandura believed people influence their environments and behaviors in goal-oriented, purposeful ways via foresight, self-regulation, and self-reflection. Bandura identified four conditions observational learning requires: *attention* to another's action; *retention*/remembering the action; *reproduction*/ability to reproduce the action; *motivation* to reproduce it. Bandura said learning could transpire without immediate behavioral changes, and learning and demonstration are separate events. Unlike behaviorists requiring demonstration to prove learning, Bandura admitted the internal states of knowledge, ideas, values, and other abstract cognitive schemes. He said students may not demonstrate learning without motivation.

## SELF-EFFICACY

Within his social cognitive theory, Bandura identified four interrelated processes that influence motivation and achieving goals: self-observation, self-evaluation, self-reaction, and self-efficacy. He coined and defined the term **self-efficacy** as people's individual beliefs in and/or judgments of their ability for accomplishing specific tasks. What an individual believes he or she can achieve under certain conditions, using his or her skills, equals that person's self-efficacy for that particular situation or activity. The more self-efficacy a person experiences about a challenging task, the more persistence and effort he or she will devote to it, making that individual more likely to succeed. Bandura explained that self-efficacy "refers to beliefs in one's capabilities to organize and execute the courses of action required to manage prospective situations." Others (Lunenburg, 2011) have characterized self-efficacy as a "task-specific version of self-esteem." People's motivation and ability to learn, as well as their subsequent performance, are influenced by self-efficacy: they frequently limit what they try to learn and perform to tasks they believe they will be able to accomplish. People are not motivated to attempt tasks they feel unequal to by ability and experience, but are motivated to learn and perform tasks for which they have high self-efficacy.

## FUNDAMENTAL ELEMENTS OF BANDURA'S SELF-EFFICACY THEORY

According to Bandura, **self-efficacy theory** is founded on the idea that people's beliefs of how effective they can be, goes on to affect their motivation and performance and on the principle that people will more likely engage in activities for which they have higher self-efficacy, less likely in those for which they have lower self-efficacy. Since people's behaviors act out their original beliefs/expectations, self-efficacy becomes a self-fulfilling prophecy.

Three dimensions wherein self-efficacy judgments are measured are:

- **Magnitude**: Whether a person feels a specific task is easy, medium, or difficult. For example, one might consider class assignments and tests or workplace tasks easy or hard.
- **Strength**: How convinced one is one can succeed at different difficulty levels. For example, one considers how confident one is one can succeed and excel at school/work tasks.
- **Generality**: The extent to which one's expectation of success can be generalized across different situations. Some authors (Redmond/Schmidt, 2014) quote Mahatma Gandhi, reflecting the theory's concept that self-efficacy influences motivation for learning: "If I have the belief that I can do it, I shall surely acquire the capacity to do it even if I may not have it at the beginning."

## FIVE BASIC HUMAN CAPABILITIES THAT ENABLE SELF-DETERMINATION

The five basic human capabilities that enable self-determination include:

- Ability to **symbolize** enables people to give life meaning, structure, continuity, and save information for future reference, allowing them to model observed behaviors.
- **Forethought** enables people to motivate, direct, and regulate actions by setting challenges and goals, plan actions and alternatives, and thus anticipate consequences before acting.
- **Vicarious learning** enables people to learn new behaviors without having to learn through trial and error by actually performing them first. They can observe others, code their observations symbolically, and use these to guide future activities, avoiding the risks of costly, even fatal errors.
- **Self-regulatory mechanisms** entail how consistently and accurately people observe and monitor their own choices, actions, and attributions; how they evaluate these; and their tangible reactions to their own behaviors. These determine how much and in what ways people engage in processes of self-regulation, which enable them to learn from their experiences and change their future behaviors accordingly.
- **Self-reflection** enables people to consider their experiences and behaviors, make sense of these, explore their own self-beliefs and cognitions, evaluate their actions and themselves, and then change their ensuing thinking and behavior based on these evaluations.

## EVALUATING SELF-EFFICACY

Information sources for evaluating self-efficacy include:

- Bandura identified **performance outcomes** (negative or positive past experiences) as most influential to decrease or increase self-efficacy. While Bandura said mastery experiences give the most "authentic evidence" of ability to succeed, enabling belief in personal competence, he also noted subsequently overcoming failures with conviction can motivate persistence in situations perceived as "achievable challenges."
- **Vicarious experiences** of others' performances (modeling) can inform people's developing high/low self-efficacy through comparing their own competence with others'. Workplace mentoring programs demonstrate this in people's encouragement by the success of others with similar skills. Weight loss/smoking cessation programs show people's discouragement from observing others' failures as well as encouragement from their successes.

- **Social/verbal persuasion**, while less powerful than performance outcomes, is influential. Positivity (e.g., "I believe in you; you can do it") increases effort; negativity (e.g., "I'm disappointed; I thought you could do better") engenders self-doubt, decreasing success probabilities.
- **Physiological feedback** (emotional arousal), the least powerful, influences self-efficacy (e.g., a racing heartbeat, sweating, and other anxiety symptoms when taking a test or making a speech undermine self-efficacy, while greater comfort raises self-efficacy).

## PROCESSES FOR EVALUATING SELF-EFFICACY

According to self-efficacy theory, three processes that people use to interpret their self-efficacy are:

- **Analysis of task requirements**: a person's judgment of what is required to perform a task
- **Attributional analysis of experience**: why a person thinks he or she performed a task at a certain level
- **Assessment of personal and situational resources or constraints**: the personal and situational factors a person identifies as being involved in performing a specific task. For example, a person might consider his or her level of skill for performing the task and/or how much effort was available for him or her to expend to accomplish the task, as personal factors. As situational factors, the person might consider such things as other demands that were competing with performing a particular task.

Some self-efficacy theorists (Gist & Mitchell, 1992) describe these assessment processes as interacting with the four factors involved in developing self-efficacy (performance outcomes/experiences, vicarious experiences/modeling, social/verbal persuasion, and physiological feedback). This interaction determines the level of self-efficacy, which then directly determines the results.

## DEVELOPMENTAL DISABILITIES

Developmental disabilities are legally defined as disabilities having onsets before the age of 18 years. Hence any disability a child has at birth or incurs before age 18 is considered developmental. Developmental disabilities include genetic syndromes, physical disabilities, behavioral disorders, and cognitive disabilities. Learning disabilities are cognitive, but distinct from intellectual disability, though these may coexist. Children with normal intelligence/ adaptive functioning otherwise can have a number of specific learning disabilities. The international term *dyslexia* describes a specific learning disability with reading, including difficulty processing language symbols; perceiving printed letters and words incorrectly/backwards; confusing similar-looking letters; trouble recognizing and decoding printed words and with reading comprehension. The international term *dysgraphia* describes difficulty composing written language. The international term *dyscalculia* describes difficulty recognizing, following, and copying numbers and number sequences and difficulty performing basic math operations like addition, subtraction, multiplication, and division. DSM-5 TR (2022) combines reading disorders, disorders of written expression, mathematics disorders, and learning disorders not otherwise specified (NOS) into Specific Learning Disorder (with codes specifying each area's deficit types) because they commonly occur together. Central auditory processing disorder impairs the receptive ability to understand, remember, organize, and manipulate the spoken language one hears.

## CONSIDERATIONS FOR TR/RT

TRSs minimize extraneous sensory stimuli; structure activities with defined spaces and limited numbers of participants; and sequence activities socially from individual and cooperative, like walking, to intergroup, like competitive team games. They may use behavioral techniques like lead-up activities, learning cues, reinforcement, structure, consistency, routine, and baseline behavior documentation to promote internally motivated, independent behaviors. They include goal-setting, prioritizing, and time management in leisure education experiences to help teen/young adult client transitions to adult and employee responsibilities. TRSs provide opportunities to develop motivation for continuing group experiences and physical activity, self-esteem, social skills, and friendship through cooperative initiatives, games, and adventure challenge education. TRSs may need to use visual, oral/auditory, and tactile cues when giving instructions and safety precautions to clients with reading and writing disabilities. Equipment with brightly marked boundaries, varying textures, and contrasting sounds and colors helps clients discriminate foreground objects vs. background surfaces. TRSs improve client spatial awareness, laterality, coordination, and directionality through movement exploration and balance activities. They compensate for part-whole dissociation with whole-task observation/completion before part performance and overlearning through repetition.

## INTELLECTUAL DISABILITIES

Intellectual disability, updated to Intellectual Developmental Disorder (IDD) in the DSM-5 TR, can be caused by various genetic syndromes, such as Down syndrome, Lesch-Nyhan syndrome, Turner syndrome, Rett syndrome, Prader-Willi syndrome, etc.; anoxia/hypoxia (oxygen deprivation) at birth; traumatic brain injury; and serious illnesses (e.g., encephalitis, meningitis, rheumatic fever, scarlet fever). IDD is diagnosed by two dimensions: intellectual ability/IQ and adaptive functioning. Historically, only IQ scores were considered; however, this limited people's opportunities and accomplishments. Whereas older versions of the DSM included IQ scores in its IDD diagnostic criteria, the DSM-5 TR (2022) omits them from the diagnostic criteria to prevent overemphasis on intelligence scores for defining overall ability. Ability to function in daily life is more important for developing treatment plans and independent/supported living. Adaptive functioning has three domains: conceptual—knowledge, memory, reasoning, language, reading, writing, and math skills; social—interpersonal communication skills, ability to make and keep friends, social judgment, empathy; and practical—personal care, work skills and responsibilities, money management, school/work organization, and recreational skills.

## ROLE OF TR/RT

For clients with IDD, TR **interventions** focus on decision making; balanced leisure lifestyles; developing, selecting, and using leisure skills and resources; participating in age-appropriate activities; community inclusion; ADLs and self-care; physical wellbeing; communication; environmental awareness; personal and community safety skills; and developing functional skills basic to leisure experiences. TR/RT protocols concentrate on remediating leisure skill deficits and cognitive behaviors. Leisure education applies interventions to remediate behavioral, social, and communication deficits and provides opportunities to participate, facilitating involvement recognition and feedback to promote self-initiated leisure functioning. Acquiring expected social behaviors, practicing verbal and nonverbal communication, understanding words with multiple meanings, and recognizing subtle nonverbal social cues are frequent areas included in social interactions provided in TR/RT for IDD clients. Sensory awareness activities, eating out, leisure education, and competition participation provide experience with appropriate dress, social greetings, restroom use, identifying directional signals and signs, making change, etc. TR/RT enables client emotional identification and expression, self-esteem, and self-improvement goals through inclusive buddy experiences, spectator events, PA, assertiveness training, and adventure/challenge activities. TR/RT improves motor fitness, performance, perceptual-motor, and motor planning skills; coordination; body rhythms; causal relationships in movement patterns; skill generalization, transfer, inclusion in community recreation; and health-related fitness and lifelong leisure skills.

## CONSIDERATIONS FOR TR/RT

Assessing client preferences in various settings is the basis for developing IDD client decision making skills, enabling successful transitions and self-initiated leisure responsibility. Environmental analysis establishes participation contexts and environmental supports, enabling TRS planning for skill generalization and transfer. Behavioral techniques helping clients perform concrete, practical tasks include task analysis, skill sequencing, shaping, chaining, modeling, demonstration, visual prompts, verbal prompts, fading, and positive reinforcement including token economies and social recognition. To encourage reciprocal communication accommodating communication deficits, TRSs should wait before speaking to allow client initiation; ask "what/how" questions, not "yes/no" questions; and not "talk down" to clients: their receptive language may exceed their expressive language. Structured environments encourage focus; practice, repetition, and activity variation promote comprehension; structured competitive games strengthen social skills. Introducing new skills early in sessions facilitates acquisition. Program-specific goals compensate for previous low/absent expectations, enabling client potential fulfillment. Similar expectations and circumstances across environments promote skill transfer. Give explicit, precise, one/two-step directions; use visual aids, hands-on learning, and repetition. Repeat trial-and-error opportunities requiring decision making. Adapt activities/equipment/materials; allow adjustment time for new situations/routine changes. Define rules and safety precautions in advance to compensate for judgment deficits. Ensure activity preparation. Teach causality by identifying antecedent-behavior-consequence (ABC).

## AUTISM SPECTRUM DISORDERS

DSM-5 TR (2022) combines the previously separated disorders of autism/autistic disorder, Asperger's disorder, childhood disintegrative disorder, and pervasive developmental disorder under **autism spectrum disorder** (ASD), reflecting scientific consensus that all these diagnoses represent levels on the spectrum of symptom severity in the same single condition. ASD is characterized by symptoms in two core domains:

- Social interaction and social communication deficits.
- Restricted, repetitive behaviors, interests, and activities (RRBs).

To diagnose ASD, symptoms in both domains must be present and not attributable to intellectual developmental disorder or global developmental delay. Individuals with ASDs have varying degrees of difficulty recognizing, understanding, and interpreting social nonverbal communications like tone of voice, facial expression, gestures, sarcasm, humor, figurative language, and nonliteral verbal expressions; expressing emotions or affection; initiating/sustaining give-and-take conversations, interactions, and relationships; and coping with unpredictable events, irregular schedules, and transitions among activities. They range from nonverbal to echolalic to highly sophisticated verbally. RBBs include rocking, hand-flapping/repetitive gestures; maintaining rigid schedules; and/or pursuing the same narrow interests and activities repeatedly and for long times.

## ROLE OF TR/RT

ASD is lifelong; therefore, so is **intervention**. Leisure and recreational skills facilitate safe, appropriate use of free time, provide bases for social interaction, and improve quality of life for ASD clients. Studies also show ASD children's language and social skills improve through play interventions. TRSs work in interdisciplinary collaborations to develop effective motor behaviors, ADLs, communicative and social interaction skills, appropriate social behaviors, appropriate environ-mental interactions, functional cognitive skills, skill generalization, community living skills, and physical wellbeing. TRSs use leisure education to help ADS clients develop skills in counting; reading directional signs; finding socially inclusive community recreation opportunities; building social acceptance, friendships, and relationships around mutual abilities and interests. TRSs also provide in-home training, including family support. TR/RT interventions decrease self-stimulatory and perseverative behaviors; improve sensory input control; develop recreation skills, appropriate social interactions, relaxation, and understanding of causality. TR experiences require attention, eye contact, cooperation, sensorimotor awareness, imitation, and expression. TRSs design experiences to redirect energy and nonfunctional behaviors to functional activity in strength areas; utilize nonlinguistic strength areas for communication; enhance self-control, decision making, and sense of accomplishment; connect consequences to actions/behaviors through visual and verbal feedback.

## CONSIDERATIONS FOR TR/RT

Make TR/RT environments, activities, locations, equipment, and times predictable and structured; maintain consistent routines. Calm, firm, predictable, consistent TRS style reassures ASD clients. Identify event sequences; prepare clients for changes. Consider bright colors, shadows as distractions. Consider whether objects can become harmful, and if unsafe places exist where clients might hide. Plan time for learning new skills 1:1 followed by group practice in every session. Plan times/places for clients to escape sensory and social overload and relax, and following "meltdowns." Ignore hand-flapping/similar behaviors that do not affect clients/others, or replace these withholding meaningful objects, etc. Use physical guidance with discretion, considering tactile-defensiveness. Visual and verbal feedback facilitates skill and meaning comprehension and transfer. Make eye contact; give directions with choices, incorporating photo/picture models. Teach various leisure skills in multiple settings toward the same goal for acquisition, generalization, and transfer. Develop specific activities/games of interest into lifetime social leisure pursuits. Incorporate client strengths into interventions to reduce challenging behaviors and increase positive interactions. Aerobic exercise on motorized equipment reduces stereotypes. Tactile and sensory feedback activities provide sustained enjoyment and reinforcement. Manage self-stimulation/self-injury using behavioral interventions. Inclusion affords natural role modeling, cooperation, built-in feedback/recognition, appropriate environmental response training, and preferred experiences.

## ATTENTION DEFICIT/HYPERACTIVITY DISORDER (ADHD)

**ADHD** is divided diagnostically into two domains: inattention and hyperactivity/impulsivity. The DSM-5 TR (APA, 2022) includes 18 symptoms as diagnostic criteria, nine under each domain. At least six symptoms in one domain must be identified as having persisted for at least six months to diagnose ADHD in children and at least five in adults with onset before 12 years of age. In light of scientific advances, the APA has classified ADHD among neurodevelopmental disorders. In the inattention domain, individuals have difficulty focusing/concentrating and cannot maintain attention for normal durations, becoming quickly and easily distracted by other environmental stimuli. It can also be more difficult to recruit their attention initially. In the hyperactivity/impulsivity domain, individuals typically have physical difficulty sitting or standing still for long and must be constantly or very frequently active. Even when sitting and watching TV, they may feel compelled to make some movement. Impulsivity manifests in inability/difficulty with controlling impulses. Individuals may interrupt others, be unable to wait to express thoughts as they occur, and/or frequently interrupt their own activities to do something else, never completing anything.

## ALZHEIMER'S DISEASE

The most common diagnosis of dementia affecting older Americans today is Alzheimer's disease/Alzheimer's-type dementia. In recent decades, up to 90% of nursing home placements have been based on this diagnosis. Early signs are memory deficits. Forgetting short-term conversations and events progresses to forgetting long-term memories of events, locations, and people. Confusion and disorientation follow. Some sufferers wander away from home, becoming lost. Alzheimer's memory loss should not be confused with normal age-related forgetfulness. Experts say a sign of Alzheimer's is not forgetting where you put your glasses or keys, but forgetting what they are. Individuals puzzle over simple everyday tasks they often performed. They develop difficulty following events in movies. They often leave ovens or stoves turned on, making living alone risky. Judgment becomes impaired; people often confuse hot and cold, dressing or adjusting HVAC inappropriately. People frequently become extremely upset when others correct/help them. A simple early screening test is asking an individual to draw a clock face indicating a specific time. Scoring criteria include drawing a closed circle; including all numbers; placing numbers correctly; and placing hands correctly. Because many conditions mimic Alzheimer's/dementia, thorough evaluation is necessary.

## NON-ALZHEIMER'S DEMENTIA

Despite the prevalence of Alzheimer's disease, other conditions can also cause dementia (e.g., atherosclerosis and arterial blockages restrict blood flow to the brain, causing cognitive impairments). AIDS can affect the brain, causing dementia. Abuse of alcohol and other substances can cause dementia. Strokes can affect many different parts of the brain. In addition to loss of motor control, speech, language, and memory, strokes can cause dementia. Like strokes, traumatic brain injuries (TBIs) caused by blows to the head can cause damage to many parts of the brain. Some of the results include aphasia, which impairs expressive and/or receptive language and speech processing; memory loss; sensory processing deficits; motor apraxia, which impairs neurological control over various body parts/movements; and dementias. Injuries damaging the frontal and prefrontal lobes of the brain can impair executive functions like planning, organization, judgment, and critical thinking. Damage to parts of the brain regulating emotion can result in emotionally labile behavior.

## TRAUMATIC BRAIN INJURY

Traumatic brain injury (TBI), sudden injury to the brain from an external force/impact, may have varying effects depending on the severity of the TBI. TBI may be primary with injury directly to the brain or secondary from injury to other parts of the body (such as a traumatic injury to the chest). TBI may occur from falls, direct impact, anoxia, assaults (including gunshot wounds) or acceleration/deceleration injuries (such as from a motor vehicle accident). Indications of a TBI may be mild (headache, mild confusion, disorientation) to severe (unable to talk, walk, or carry out any ADLs) with most clients located somewhere along the continuum. TBI may profoundly affect a client's cognitive abilities, physical abilities, and behavioral/emotional functioning. The most common cause of TBI in general is motor vehicle accidents, but for the very young and very old, falls cause most TBIs. Adolescents and young adults often experience TBI from sports-related accidents. Clients with TBI are at high risk for substance abuse disorders, often seeking to self-medicate.

### *TR/RT CONSIDERATIONS FOR NEUROMUSCULAR IMPAIRMENTS*

TRSs must consider pain tolerance levels and behavioral symptoms like mood swings and depression as sequelae of **traumatic brain injuries (TBIs) and spinal cord injuries (SCIs)** and establish a communication system at program outset. Dysphagia (swallowing difficulty) must be considered when planning meal functions for clients with strokes, TBIs, or Parkinson's disease. SCIs limit activity, decreasing fitness and causing obesity; TRSs promote maximum caloric activity and oxygen intake through active and passive ROM and extension exercises. Lighter equipment and shorter exercise times are important for physically impaired clients. Larger areas, slower paces, and sooner rest periods for exacerbated client fatigue are indicated with mobility aid and appliance use. Strokes and TBIs affecting the right hemisphere cause slow, disorganized responses; left-hemisphere damage causes insensitive, self-centered-appearing behavior. Slow/long rehabilitation durations require TRS patience. Leisure education improves client social connections and community resource awareness. Program planning must consider parking lot, telephone, restroom, water fountain, and other support area accessibility. TRSs can use the buddy system strategically to enable clients to compensate for each other's functional deficits.

## MUSCULOSKELETAL IMPAIRMENTS

Various musculoskeletal impairments may require RT/TR interventions:

- **Osteogenesis imperfecta (OI)** is inherited, causing brittle, easily fractured bones and small stature. Depending on severity, patients may need wheelchairs. TRSs must take care when transferring and assisting to avoid fractures.
- **Osteoporosis** is bone mineral loss causing porous, brittle bones prone to fractures. It is more prevalent in the aging; Asian and Caucasian races; females; thin, small-boned individuals; and is secondary to bed rest, physical inactivity, cerebral palsy, spinal cord injuries, cancer, and cancer treatment. Pathological fractures can result from simply changing positions.
- **Spina bifida** is a birth defect caused by incomplete closure of the spinal column. Depending on spinal lesion level, symptoms range from foot weakness to paraplegia below the waist.
- **Arthritis** encompasses over 100 conditions involving joint inflammation.
- **Myasthenia gravis**, a chronic disease with flare-ups and remissions, causes progressive muscle weakness, beginning with eye/facial, jaw, and throat muscles, progressing to arm, back, abdominal, and leg muscles. Respiratory muscle involvement can be fatal.
- **Muscular dystrophies** are related genetic muscular diseases causing progressive atrophy and weakness in voluntary muscles. Duchenne, or childhood, MD is most common and severe. Daily exercise initially slows progression, but functional ability declines faster after patients require wheelchairs, in stage 5 of 8. Stage 8=bedridden.

## TR/RT SERVICES AVAILABLE

TR/RT services available to specific musculoskeletal disorders include the following:

- **Muscular dystrophy:** Children have fewer opportunities to play; adults are affected in work and social activities by degenerative processes. TR programs should enhance quality of life by improving social networks; augmenting self-control; fostering meaningful use of spare time; maintaining strength, range of motion, mobility, and fitness; and prolonging independent functioning. Muscles used for breathing and wheelchair ambulation benefit from yoga, swimming, and rhythmic breathing. Contractures are prevented by ROM activities, stretching, and flexion-extension exercises. Seated exercises help posture and strengthen muscles for ADLs and wheelchair transfers. Leisure education supports adjustment to bed rest and wheel-chair use.
- **Arthritis**: Chronic pain and extent of joint damage and involvement determine TR participation. Swimming, cycling, stretching, relaxation, creative movement, and target/throwing games encourage full-ROM movement and prevent extended weight-bearing durations. Leisure education aids inclusive wellness options awareness, adherence to weight management and activity routines, new leisure skills, and adaptation to lifestyle changes.
- **Osteoporosis**: Passive ROM exercise and tilt-tables can slow calcium loss rates. Resistance/weight-bearing exercises like yoga and walking help ambulatory clients.

- **Myasthenia gravis**: TR maintains breathing capacity, allows rest periods, and avoids prolonged walking or standing through swimming; social and cognitive (e.g., journaling) experiences further self-control and expression, and combat depression.

## NERVOUS SYSTEM IMPAIRMENTS

**Cerebral palsy (CP)**, the most common childhood disability, impairs the brain's ability to control and coordinate the muscles. Limb involvement can be monoplegia/one limb; hemiplegia/both limbs on one side; diplegia/lower limbs with mild upper-limb involvement; triplegia/three limbs; paraplegia/lower limbs; or quadriplegia/four limbs. Symptoms include spasticity, with muscle hypertension, contractions, and an uncontrolled stretch reflex, causing postural deviations; athetosis, with constant uncontrollable, involuntary, unpredictable, purposeless movements, mitigated by relaxation; ataxia, with impaired coordination and balance; rigidity, with stiffness and impaired stretch reflex; tremors, or uncontrolled, involuntary, rhythmic motions, randomly or upon initiating movement; and "mixed." **Seizure disorders** are episodes of abnormal brain activity causing sudden changes in consciousness/behavior and involuntary motor activity. Absence/petit mal seizures involve brief lapses in consciousness. Tonic-clonic/grand mal seizures involve rigid, then jerky movements, loss of consciousness, and sleep. Atonic/drop seizures involve momentary consciousness lapse and loss of postural tone. **Multiple sclerosis** destroys myelin sheaths protecting the brain and spinal cord, replacing them with scar tissue interrupting nerve impulse transmission. MS can be benign or relapsing-remitting, progressive, or combinations of the two. Symptoms and disability vary widely.

> **Review Video: Multiple Sclerosis (MS)**
> Visit mometrix.com/academy and enter code: 417355

## ROLE OF TR/RT

TRSs can help **cerebral palsy** patients tolerate longer movement periods with less tension, fatigue, and overstimulation through weight lifting, water aerobics, and individualized relaxation and stress management programs. Swimming, therapeutic horseback riding, cycling, and target activities incorporating balance, extension, bilateral movement, free gross motor actions, and spatial relationships can promote motor functioning. TRSs provide transportation assistance supporting family care, and leisure education and inclusion supporting educational and transition plans throughout school and adulthood. They help clients develop positive self-images and identities, fitness, proper posture, fall prevention through exercise, community resource awareness, and self-expression through creative arts, etc., as well as acquire, adapt, adjust to and use orthoses/braces and assistive devices. TRS services to clients **with seizure disorders** vary individually. Parents and doctors are often overprotective about sports/exercise participation; generally, the benefits outweigh evidence of injury/increased seizures. Helmets and supervision are required for activities risking falls like adventure/cycling. TRSs can design programs promoting progressive physical wellbeing and controlling excess environmental stimulation; mitigate stigma, social isolation, fear, stress, and lowered self-concept related to seizure disorders through education; and combine psychotherapy with camping/skiing/similar TR programs, which improves children's self-esteem. Relaxation training, creative expression, and role-playing also promote lifestyle adjustments and coping skills.

## CIRCULATORY IMPAIRMENTS

**Coronary heart disease (CHD)** is the most common acquired heart disease, including myocardial infarction (MI/heart attack), acute ischemic coronary artery disease (CAD), and atherosclerosis. CAD is caused by decreased blood supply to the heart resulting from narrowed coronary arteries. Lifestyle factors like diet and inactivity contribute to accumulation of fatty and fibrous materials that form blood clots. These obstruct coronary arteries (thrombosis), causing heart attack, or break off and travel, obstructing other arteries (embolism); in the brain, this causes stroke. Hypertension involves above-normal pressure of blood against inner blood vessel walls, taxing the heart. Hypertension can be accompanied by arteriosclerosis/artery wall hardening and/or atherosclerosis/accumulation of fatty plaques in arteries. CAD is primarily caused by atherosclerosis due to hypertension, obesity, and other lifestyle-related conditions (though some people are thin, exercise frequently, and have genetically high cholesterol). When coronary arteries supply less oxygenated blood than the heart muscle needs, heart attack ensues. Congestive heart failure, caused by fluid accumulation secondary to weak heart pumping, can result from heart valve defects, hypertension, MI, CAD, inactivity/being bedridden, and other causes. Hemophilia, a hereditary clotting factor disorder, causes excessive bleeding following injury. Anemia reduces blood's oxygen-transporting ability due to hemoglobin/red blood cell deficiency.

## CONSIDERATIONS FOR TR/RT

Cardiac functioning and damage diversity requires comprehensive approaches to recovery, preventing recurrences, and promoting general health. Assessing and rehabilitating functional capacity are treatment foci. Goals must fall within physician-set parameters. TRSs must monitor heart rate, blood pressure, oxygen saturation, respiration, perceived exertion and pain, faintness, dizziness, and nausea during interventions, and consider environmental effects on client vital signs, including temperature, humidity, wind chill, and elevation. They must be familiar with the effects of cardiac pharmaceuticals on exercise responses. Health promotion and education concentrate on reducing risk factors through lifestyle adjustments like controlling blood pressure, cholesterol, and weight. TRSs as team members incorporate interventions promoting self-regulation and address hidden disabilities. During client hospitalization, TRSs offer passive interventions and use techniques for adapting activities to prevent dangerous cardiac loads. They raise awareness of lifestyle-leisure relationships. Also, they teach self-monitoring of heart rate, blood pressure, and diet, promoting caregiver/family support. As client exercise tolerance progresses, TRSs support inpatient-to-outpatient program transitions and community reintegration and promote compliance with medication and lifestyle regimes required for lifetime risk-factor reduction.

## RESPIRATORY IMPAIRMENTS

Respiratory impairments include chronic bronchitis, involving bronchial inflammation and mucus; emphysema, wherein the lungs' alveoli/air sacs are irreversibly destroyed; asthma, involving chronic airway inflammation, narrowing, obstruction, and sensitivity; cystic fibrosis (CF), a genetic disorder causing abnormally sticky, thick mucus that obstructs breathing, impedes digestion, and causes malnutrition; and tuberculosis, a bacterial infection causing inflammation and lung damage. TRSs conduct rehabilitation programs, preserving physical capacity and emotional adjustment to chronic illness; evaluate and report functional levels in education and treatment plans; implement leisure education; facilitate community reintegration; promote healthy lifestyles; encourage physical activity moderation, appropriate warmup, and sometimes medication before exercise; consider weather, pollution, and other environmental conditions; and teach pursed-lip and diaphragmatic breathing exercises and relaxation techniques to enhance expiration capacity. Aerobics, swimming, cycling, walking, and jogging aid cardiorespiratory fitness, chest muscles, and cough reflex; weight training, tennis, and golf build shoulder and abdominal muscles; blowing exercises/activities help expel residual air. TRSs must consider real/perceived activity barriers: fearing attacks can prevent activity, promoting stress and overweight, triggering attacks. Leisure education promotes lifestyle changes and risk reduction; resource awareness promotes adaptive equipment use; social engagement, spirituality experiences, and humor provide coping mechanisms and distractions.

## DIABETES

Clients with primary or secondary diabetes diagnoses are most likely to have TRSs implement health promotion and education programs. Type 1 diabetics are usually normal weight, Type 2 more often overweight. Treating both includes evaluating and monitoring diet, exercise, blood sugar levels, medication(s), and secondary complications. For obese clients, TRSs design health promotion and education activities promoting physical activity, good nutrition, weight management, and psychosocial support and wellbeing; additionally, emphasize proper nutrition need and value, regular exercise habits, and time management skills; and teach stress management and relaxation techniques promoting coping and risk behavior self-control. They help overweight/lean clients adopt and maintain low-fat, high-carbohydrate diets in smaller, more frequent meals, maintaining consistent blood sugar levels and regulating weight. Education programs center on managing blood sugar levels before, during, and after meals and exercise to avoid complications, and managing lifestyle changes. TRSs monitor heart rates and blood pressure to help clients prevent/identify heart disease. Health promotion helps identify and reduce stressors triggering poor eating behaviors. Leisure resource awareness eliminates PA obstacles and identifies enjoyable options. With younger clients, family education and support are key. Social experiences increase self-confidence, promoting continuing engagement through shared interests. TRS-provided assertion, values clarification, and problem-solving experiences promote client responsibility.

## VISUAL IMPAIRMENT

For clients with visual impairment, TRSs help establish accessible environments and encourage participation in PA and sports for sensory stimulation, community resource access, social experiences, weight management, and self-confidence. TR fosters resource awareness and leisure skill development. Therapists promote PA in the com-munity and at home for older clients; offer health promotion and educational experiences encouraging self-directed participation; create safe environments; and support training in balance, spatial awareness, and other necessary basic skills. TRSs create accessible opportunities and environments when providing direct services by adapting equipment and activities; orienting clients; serving as seeing guides; and creating accessibility using various auditory, tactile, and kinesthetic stimuli. TRSs give clients orientation and mobility (O&M) training, facilitating access to leisure experiences. They help other service providers and caregivers market and deliver services. Fitness, movement exploration, and aquatics activities help clients relax; develop self- and postural awareness relative to others and environmental objects; and monitor their expressions and movements. Leisure education introduces clients to alternative reading devices for self-directed experiences. Early intervention using play groups affords young children sensory stimulation, movement exploration, environmental obstacle adaptation, other-aware-ness, and social interaction, increasing access and participation.

### TEACHING STRATEGIES AND TECHNIQUES

Activities TRSs design include physical guidance; guided recovery; whole-part-whole instruction; audible targets; marked boundaries; sound-source devices; tactile modeling; demonstration; audio recordings; Braille; large print; paired auditory and touch stimuli; boundaries; hand and foot placements; and using audible goals, voice commands and varying textures to identify starting, turning, and stopping points. To teach skills, they may use task analysis; concise, clear directions; touch with permission; slower activity paces to accommodate mobility aids and objects; glare and shadow control to improve visual awareness in the partially sighted; multisensory exploration of physical boundaries; light variations and smells for identifying and remembering locations; rails/guide ropes marking trails/paths; balls in phosphorescent colors; and removing unnecessary environmental objects and noises. In orientation and mobility training, TRSs may use compass/clock faces to describe object locations; alphabet letters for entry-exit route reference

54

points; verbally announce their name and approach/departure; identify client residual vision and best conversational position; help clients identify hazards, memorize warning signals, and practice emergency procedures. Clients may use laser canes, guide dogs, and/or sighted partners/guides during activities.

## HEARING IMPAIRMENTS

Clients with hearing impairments vary in hearing acuity, ability to benefit from hearing aids, and dependence on vision and touch for environmental and social interactions. Hearing loss secondary to semicircular canal damage includes balance disruption. Preferred client communication methods influence leisure patterns. TRSs control lighting conditions and environmental distractions, which influence the effectiveness of oral and manual communication methods. For example, wearing clothing with dark solid colors facilitates signing and finger-spelling. Leisure experiences provided by TRSs afford clients with hearing losses expressive and creative outlets, relaxation, tension relief, venues for social interaction, physical activity, sensory development, and improve their functional independence, self-determination, decision-making skills, problem-solving skills, spontaneity, and wellbeing. Because sports depend less on verbal communication than many other leisure activities, deaf people seem to experience less constraint playing sports. Deaf identity, attitudes, social competence, and use of varying communication methods contribute to challenges clients encounter in inclusive recreation activities. TRSs therefore play vital roles in establishing recreational opportunities with family and friends. They increase positive attitudes and social experiences, and decrease obstacles, through providing leisure education and participation in ongoing communication training.

### INTERVENTION STRATEGIES

Stand in client view; allow clients to move to view you. Keep your mouth empty and lips visible. Be aware of sunshine, glare, shade, and shadows. Only give directions while clients face you. Speak to clients, not interpreters. Minimize background noise. Write down words as needed; repeat short sentences. Speak in normal tones, clearly but naturally; emphasize meaning and feeling using facial expressions and gestures. Model skills being developed. Introduce movement patterns using physical guidance and guided discovery; enable clients to view others performing skills. Train clients to detect dangerous circumstances visually. Use visual start/stop cues. Demonstrate fast/slow directions for clients' visual discrimination. Demonstrate terms with multiple meanings. Instruct clients to widen support bases and lower centers of gravity to compensate for unsteady balance. Place mirrors to aid client movement/skill development. Enhance client self-awareness through relaxation experiences. Include rhythm activities to help clients develop motor skills to support poise in social settings. To help clients discriminate immediate sounds from background interference, teach them to focus on your instructions and cues. To assess client comprehension and compliance capacity, request demonstration/feedback; ask questions. Prepare multiple alternatives to sustain attention in children needing stronger guidance/easily distracted.

## SCHIZOPHRENIA

Schizophrenia impairs the ability to perceive, process, and respond to reality. Thoughts, perceptions, emotions, and interactions become dissociated from each other and disorganized. Symptoms include delusions, hallucinations, loose associations, incoherence, lack of insight, distractibility, flattened or inappropriate affect, extreme inactivity or hyperactivity, bizarre repetitive behaviors, impaired social skills, social withdrawal, and apathy or lack of interest and enjoyment in relationships or activities. Helpful treatments include combined antipsychotic medication and group psychosocial therapy; behaviorist social reinforcement techniques; and family education and therapy to reduce home stressors. TR/RT interventions include family leisure education; reducing motor behavior symptoms and social withdrawal and underlying stressors;

and structured exercise groups, recreation experiences, and social interactions. Intense, emotional group interactions should be avoided as threatening. TR/RT can increase attention span; cognitive, language, and decision-making skills; and learning and following rules. Recreation experiences serve as coping mechanisms to help clients with stressful situations without withdrawing into isolation and delusion. Increased physical activity seems to aid client emotional expression and management. TR/RT may also support work-related stress management.

## MOOD AND ANXIETY DISORDERS

**Depression** involves feelings of overwhelming sadness, helplessness, hopelessness, and suicidal ideations to escape the misery. Individuals with depressive disorders withdraw socially, lose interest in their usual activities and relationships, become apathetic, and often neglect personal hygiene. They may have insomnia or sleep too much. A common process in depression that leads to suicide is the perception that one's options or solutions progressively decrease until they have no other choice. **Mania** involves excessive energy, hyperactivity, unrealistic feelings of power and invincibility, irritability, and insomnia. Patients experience flight of ideas; may talk too fast and excessively; and go on binges of activity without sleeping for days. **Bipolar disorder** involves dramatic, cyclical swings between mania and depression. Because bipolar disorder has strong familial and physiological components, treatment often includes mood-stabilizing medications. Among many types of **anxiety disorders**, generalized anxiety disorder involves excessive worry over everything, disrupting normal life. **Panic disorder** involves periodic, sudden, intense anxiety attacks with physiological symptoms. **Phobic disorders** involve persistent abnormal fears of specific things, events, or situations. **Obsessive-compulsive disorder** involves obsessive thoughts and compulsive actions.

> **Review Video: Different Types of Anxiety Disorders**
> Visit mometrix.com/academy and enter code: 366760

## TR/RT INTERVENTIONS

Physical activity stimulates mood-stabilizing neurotransmitter production and enhances stress-management coping skills. Research finds physically active people less likely to develop depression. TRSs encourage inactive clients gradually to develop more active lifestyles, increase aerobic fitness, and develop individualized fitness plans. Distorted self-concept, lowered self-esteem, learned helplessness, and societal stigma regarding psychological disorders are common among clients with emotional disorders; TR/RT builds self-esteem and improves client perspectives and attitudes toward themselves. When TRSs lead activity-based programs, they can help clients explore the origins of their lowered self-esteem and effectively raise client self-esteem by choosing and sequencing activities that are positively reinforcing to clients. TR/RT programs incorporating creative expression along with PA can relieve/reduce anxiety. TR/RT programs incorporating behavioral techniques use conditioning and systematic desensitization to decrease anxiety. Cognitive therapies teach coping skills via stress management, biofeedback, relaxation techniques, assertion therapy, etc. Humanistic values clarification approaches help clients identify their most satisfying leisure experiences, for which TRSs can then teach necessary knowledge and skills. For clients beginning mood-stabilizing pharmacotherapy, during the 2–3 weeks until medication takes effect, TRSs use structured activities to help manic clients channel their energy into meaningful activities and address depressed clients' limited motivation with short-term, success-oriented activities.

## SUBSTANCE ABUSE AND ADDICTION DISORDERS

Abuse of alcohol and other drugs/substances cause more illnesses, disabilities, and deaths than all other preventable health conditions. Heavy alcohol and drug use are associated with anxiety and depressive disorders. Clients seeking substance abuse treatment have higher incidence of additional psychiatric disorders. Substance-related disorders are more prevalent among criminal offenders, homeless persons, HIV-positive individuals, people with antisocial personality disorders, and children of substance abusers. Chronic substance abuse impairs physical and psychological functioning. Since alcohol and drug use transpire during leisure time, researchers find users expect alcohol/drugs to enable and enhance their leisure experiences. Alcohol and many other drugs are physically and psychologically addictive, making it extremely difficult for addicts to cease use due to the horrible withdrawal symptoms they experience. Moreover, when personality dysfunctions originally prompted substance abuse, if not remediated, they will inevitably trigger relapse. TRSs help clients replace substances with healthy alternatives producing similar feelings and help them develop stress-management, problem-solving, and decision-making skills. They support client development of feelings of competence, mastery, and control during recovery. TRSs help clients learn to structure and manage free time and choose leisure experiences promoting self-esteem, self-efficacy, and trusting relationships.

## ROLE OF TR/RT

Throughout their interventions, TRSs serve as role models for clients recovering from substance abuse. They facilitate client relaxation and playfulness as they also encourage clients to develop lifestyles that will afford them better health and management of substance use. To begin, TRSs assess clients' individual personality and social needs. They address self-defeating client behaviors (e.g., low tolerance thresholds and dependency). They work with clients to help them develop self-control, cooperative behaviors, communication skills, and trusting relationships. They assist clients in learning to function more independently, develop support networks, and improve their physical wellbeing. Effective TR/RT supports other therapy in promoting abstinence and preventing relapse. Relapse prevention is aided when TRSs help clients develop, practice, and incorporate leisure options they perceive as self-governing, challenging, and rewarding into their value systems. TRSs collaborate with clients in implementing structured, success-oriented leisure and recreation experiences. Throughout this process, they confront clients' typical behaviors of denial, impulsivity, attention-seeking, and manipulation. Through interdisciplinary practice, TRSs can collaborate with other practitioners in structured family programming and family therapy settings, benefiting clients by educating family, reducing home/family stress, addressing dysfunctional family dynamics, and engaging family support and participation in client recovery.

## ASSESSMENT TOOLS

### IMPACT OF TR/RT ON SOCIAL SKILLS AND ATTITUDES

The **Measurement of Social Empowerment and Trust** (SET, Wittman, 1991) tests how clients' perceived social attitudes and skills have changed due to participation in a TR/RT treatment program or adventure/challenge course. A self-report assessment for adults and adolescents with moderate to no cognitive impairment, this test includes five subscales:

- Bonding/cohesion: how much one respondent sees oneself as connected with a group
- Empowerment: perception of one's ability to influence people and events
- Self-awareness: ability to identify one's own feelings
- Self-affirmations: ability to express one's beliefs and goals
- Awareness of others: awareness of others and trust in them

Statements for respondents to agree/disagree with include that one feels accepted by others, understands how one's actions affect others, and feels one currently can get along with a group. Another instrument by Wittman (1987) is the **Cooperation and Trust Scale (CAT).** Administered to adolescents in a summer adventure program, this self-report scale is appropriate for clients with high cognitive function to measure their perceived trust and cooperation levels.

## PSYCHOLOGICAL STATUS, SOCIAL SKILLS, AND BEHAVIORS

The **Comprehensive Evaluation in Recreational Therapy–Psychiatric/Behavioral** (CERT–Psych/R) is among the oldest standardized tests still currently in use. Although originally developed for use with adults who were diagnosed with psychiatric disorders, TR/RT experts find it equally applicable for assessment with adults and youth without psychiatric diagnoses. It has been administered in large state facilities and acute care centers. Some TR/RT experts believe it is more appropriate for use with clients receiving more long-term inpatient services. The purpose of this test is the identification and evaluation of client behaviors related to applying appropriate social skills that will enable them to integrate into society successfully. It utilizes an observational checklist. It is divided into three areas of performance:

- **General** (appearance, attendance, attitude toward therapy, etc.)
- **Individual performance** (attention span, strength, endurance, performance in free and organized activities, frustration tolerance, decision-making skills, hostility expressed, etc.)
- **Group performance** (group conversation, leadership ability in groups, responses to group structure, etc. The CERT–PB can be used repeatedly following each session/treatment setting for documenting interactions.)

## ASSESSMENT TOOLS FOR FUNCTIONAL LEISURE SKILLS
## FACTR

The **Functional Assessment of Characteristics for Therapeutic Recreation, Revised** (FACTR; Peterson, Dunn & Carruthers, 1983; FACTR–R, revised by Burlingame) was originally designed for adult VA hospital patients, including those receiving acute hospitalization, rehabilitation, psychiatric, geriatric, and other services. It is applicable to most populations for use as an initial screening instrument. Its purpose is to assess basic functional skills, to determine whether a client qualifies for TR/RT services, and to identify in which areas the client is most likely to improve from receiving TR/RT services. It is divided into three domains:

- Physical: ambulation, general coordination, vision, hearing
- Cognitive: attention, orientation, concentration, long-term memory, receptive language
- Emotional/social: functioning in dyads, small groups, competition, conflicts or arguments

The assessment data are collected using observation and chart review. The Functional Fitness Assessment for Adults over 60 Years (Osness et al, 1996) is designed to determine functional abilities, compared to age and sex norms, of seniors with limited disabilities for performing ADLs. It tests six physical function areas: body composition, flexibility, agility/dynamic balance, coordination, strength, and endurance.

## CERT-PD

The **Comprehensive Evaluation in Recreational Therapy–Physical Disabilities** (CERT–PD; Parker, 1988) is an assessment that uses an observational checklist. It is intended for evaluating adult clients in rehabilitation programs. Its purpose is to establish baseline levels of client functional skills needed for leisure activities. It is divided into eight areas of functioning: (1) gross motor function (weight bearing, neck control, lower extremity movement ability), (2) fine motor function (manual movement ability, manual movement endurance), (3) locomotion (ambulation ability, wheelchair maneuverability, transfer ability), (4) motor skills (gross motor coordination, fine motor coordination, reaction time), (5) sensory (visual acuity, depth perception, ocular pursuit, auditory acuity), (6) cognition (attention span, memory, orientation, judgment, decision-making ability), (7) communication (verbal receptive skills, verbal expressive skills, reading receptive skills, written expressive skills), and (8) behavior (social interaction skills, adjustment to disability, frustration tolerance level, displays of emotion).

## ASSESSMENT TOOLS FOR INDIVIDUALS WITH INTELLECTUAL DISABILITY

The **General Recreation Screening Tool** (GRST; Burlingame, 1988) was designed for evaluating adults placed in intermediate care facilities for the intellectually disabled. It applies to developmental levels from 0–6 months up to 7–10 years. The purpose of this screening tool is to identify general developmental levels of functioning in 18 skill areas associated with leisure activity: (1) gross motor skills; (2) fine motor skills; (3) eye-hand coordination; (4) play behavior; (5) play structure; (6) language use; (7) language comprehension; (8) understanding of numbers; (9) use of objects; (10) following directions; (11) problem solving; (12) attending behavior; (13) possessions; (14) emotional control; (15) imitation play; (16) people skills; (17) music; and (18) stories and drama. The method of assessment is observational. The Recreation Early Development Screening Tool (REDS; Burlingame, 1988) is one of the few TR/RT assessment instruments available for adults with profound intellectual and severe developmental disabilities whose functioning is below the one-year-old level. Its purpose is to determine developmental levels from 0–1 month up to 8–12 months. Using observational methods, it measures five areas: gross motor, fine motor, sensory, and social/cognition.

## LONG-TERM CARE MINIMUM DATA SET

MDS stands for **Minimum Data Set,** whose full name is the Long-Term Care Minimum Data Set. This is a standardized tool designed for long-term healthcare facilities whose residents receive Medicare or Medicaid benefits, to conduct primary screenings and assessments of resident health status. Pursuant to OBRA (Omnibus Budget Reconciliation Act) legislation, passed in 1987 and effective by 1990, the Centers for Medicare and Medicaid Services (CMS) require all US states to report long-term care facility resident outcomes. In addition to assessing health status, the MDS is a tool for long-term care facilities to determine and obtain reimbursement from Medicare and Medicaid for services to residents covered by these programs and a tool for facilitating quality improvement in long-term healthcare facilities. It is used for assessment five days after resident admission, again at specified intervals, and whenever changes in services occur. It includes sections for documenting resident activity preferences and TR/RT results. TR/RT services provided by qualified CTRSs are ordered by physicians for residents as part of their active treatment. Facilities report data using online retrieval systems for direct service provider reimbursements.

## FUNCTIONAL INDEPENDENCE MEASURE (FIM)

FIM stands for **Functional Independence Measure**. This assessment measures a client's level of functional ability. Its score indicates the degree of disability and how much care is required. The FIM has advantages of being quick to administer, suitable for group administration, and applicable across different disciplines. Rehabilitation programs/centers commonly employ the FIM; it is the assessment most frequently used in America in the rehabilitation field. As a client's level of disability changes in severity during rehabilitation, therapists can use FIM data to track these changes and analyze the results and effectiveness of rehabilitation. The FIM contains 18 items, including 13 motor tasks and 5 cognitive tasks related to activities of daily living (ADLs). Each item is assessed by identifying one of seven levels. The two highest levels indicate independence; the lower five represent progressively greater need for assistance. The FIM's 18 areas are: eating, grooming, bathing, upper-body dressing, lower-body dressing, toileting, bladder management, bowel management, bed-to-chair transfer, toilet transfer, shower transfer, locomotion (ambulatory or wheelchair), stairs, cognitive comprehension, expression, social interaction, problem-solving, and memory.

## EXAMPLES OF DESCRIPTIONS USED

The Functional Independence Measure (FIM) measures the levels at which an individual functions in 18 dimensions of daily living activities/self-care. When a TRS is certified as a FIM Assessor, he or she is responsible for assessing clients in all 18 areas of the FIM. TRSs frequently focus on the FIM areas of cognitive comprehension, expression, and social interaction. In a FIM functional description of comprehension, the TRS would indicate the client understood best when the TRS (a) spoke to the client; (b) wrote, gestured, or used sign language; (c) used an equal combination of speech and writing/gesture/signing; or (d) the client's best mode of comprehension could not be assessed. A functional description of expression would indicate the client communicated mostly by (a) talking; (b) writing, gesturing, or signing; (c) an equal combination of (a) and (b); or (d) the client's mode of expression could not be assessed. Identifying one of seven levels at which a client functions in each area assessed gives more detail about specifically what assistance the client needs to perform each activity.

## SEVEN LEVELS OF FUNCTIONAL ABILITY

- Level 7 = Complete independence.
- Level 6 = Modified independence.
- Level 5 = Client requires supervision or setup.
- Level 4 = Minimal contact assistance: Client performs 75% or more of the task.
- Level 3 = Moderate assistance: Client performs 50–74% of the task.
- Level 2 = Maximum assistance: Client performs 25–49% of the task.
- Level 1 = Dependent/total assistance: Client performs <25% of the task.
- Level 0 = No activity occurs.

## ON THE SOCIAL INTERACTION SCALE:

- 7 = Client interacts appropriately with others 100% of the time.
- 6 = Occasional inappropriate behavior, but self-corrects; or medication required (antipsychotic, antianxiety, antidepressant, etc.).
- 5 = Client only needs behavioral supervision under unfamiliar or stressful conditions, less than 10% of the time.
- 4 = Client interacts appropriately 75–90% of the time.
- 3 = Client interacts appropriately 50–74% of the time.
- 2= Client interacts appropriately 25–49% of the time.
- 1 = Client interacts appropriately less than 25% of the time.
- 0 = Client never interacts appropriately/does not interact. Inappropriate behavior observations include: non-interactive/withdrawn; excessive crying/laughing; loud, abusive, foul language; temper tantrums; physical attacks; requiring restraints for safety.

## LEISURE COMPETENCE MEASURE

The Leisure Competence Measure (LCM) is defined as an "assessment summary" rather than an actual assessment. It is modeled on the Functional Independence Measure (FIM). A standardized instrument, the LCM is designed to measure client outcomes. Like the FIM, it divides skills into seven levels, ranging from total independence to complete dependence, with each level in between representing progressive amounts of assistance that the client needs to perform each skill. The LCM has the advantage of being adaptable to administer in nearly any setting. It includes eight subsections:

- Leisure awareness
- Leisure attitude
- Leisure skills
- Cultural/social behaviors
- Interpersonal skills
- Community integration skills
- Social contact
- Community participation.

The first six of these subscales indicate the capacities of the client, while the seventh and eighth measure the actual performance of the client. The seventh and eighth subscales may be utilized as screening tools to ascertain whether the client needs services.

## GLOBAL ASSESSMENT OF FUNCTIONING (GAF)

GAF stands for Global Assessment of Functioning. It is considered the most often used scale for assessing impairment in patients with psychiatric disorders. Mental health and social work practitioners use it during patient or caregiver interviews to make global assessments, probably more often than any other similar instruments. According to the APA, it is especially helpful as a single measure for tracking individual patients' clinical progress in global terms. The GAF was Axis V of the DSM-IV-TR (APA, 2000); however, its successor, the DSM-5, then eliminated multiaxial diagnosis and also the GAF. While critics find it too subjective, the GAF still has widespread utility among experienced practitioners who know how to use it for defining the overall psychological, social, and occupational functioning of an individual. The GAF uses a 100-point continuum of single items, from superior functioning with no symptoms (100–91) to persistent danger of harming self/others/inability to maintain minimal personal hygiene/serious suicidal act with clear intention of death (10–1). This 100-point scale is divided into ten functional ranges, though when applicable, intermediate scores are also possible.

### POINT RANGES

**100–91:** no psychiatric symptoms; superior functioning in a wide range of activities. **90–81:** minimal symptoms (occasional family arguments, mild anxiety before stressful events); good functioning in every area, wide activity range; social effectiveness, general life satisfaction. **80–71:** transient, expected reactions to stressors, like trouble concentrating following family conflict; only slight impairment in functioning, like temporary slips in school/work performance. **70–61:** some mild symptoms, like mild insomnia, anxious/depressed mood; or some functional difficulty, but functions fairly well generally; some meaningful relationships. **60–51:** moderate symptoms (occasional panic attacks); circumstantial, flat conversation; moderate functional difficulty like co-worker/family conflicts, few friends. **50–41:** serious symptoms like shoplifting frequently, obsessive-compulsive rituals, suicidal ideation; or serious functional impairment like inability to hold jobs, no friends. **40–31:** some communicative/reality-testing impairment (illogical, irrelevant, or obscure speech) or major impairment in several areas (family interactions, school or work, mood, thinking, or judgment). **30–21:** delusions, hallucinations; seriously impaired judgment/communication; cannot function in most areas. **20–11:** some danger of harming self/others or gross communication impairment; occasionally cannot maintain minimal personal hygiene. **10–1:** persistent danger of harming self/others or inability to maintain minimal personal hygiene or serious suicidal act. 0: insufficient information.

## *YMCA FITNESS ASSESSMENT*

The YMCA Fitness Testing and Assessment Manual identifies its Fitness Assessment's purposes as evaluating a person's current fitness levels, identifying his or her training needs, choosing a training regimen, motivating the individual to exercise, and evaluating a training program's effectiveness in accomplishing its goals. When scheduling assessment appointments, test-takers are advised not to drink alcohol for 24 hours prior to the test day, not to drink caffeinated beverages on the day of testing, not to smoke tobacco for two hours prior to testing, not to exercise on the testing day, not to eat any food for two hours before the tests begin, and to wear suitable exercise shoes and clothing for the assessment. One component of the YMCA Fitness Assessment is a health screening, to identify medical prohibitions against certain or all exercises; disease risks; potential medical evaluation needs; possible stress test needs; need for medical supervision in exercise programs; other special needs; and American College of Sports Medicine (ACSM) risk levels according to age and risk factors like medical conditions, symptoms, and/or diseases.

## PHYSICAL FITNESS COMPONENTS

In addition to a health screening, the YMCA Fitness Assessment includes physical fitness tests covering: standard measurements (height, weight, resting blood pressure, and heart rate), body composition, cardiovascular fitness, flexibility, muscular strength and endurance, and additional screenings/tests at local YMCA Medical Advisory Committee discretion. Height is measured to the nearest ¼-in/cm without shoes, weight to the nearest ¼-lb/kg without shoes in shorts and t-shirt. Resting heart rate is measured in upright, seated position while rested, relaxed, and comfortable, for one minute using a stethoscope. Normal resting heart rate is 50–100 beats per minute/bpm; average is 72 bpm; an aerobically fit person's rate is 50–65 bpm; an aerobically fit athlete's rate is 40–50 bpm. Resting systolic and diastolic blood pressure is measured in the same position without conversation, using a cuff, stethoscope, and sphygmomanometer. Body composition is assessed by measuring skinfolds with calipers at the abdomen, ilium, triceps, and thigh; weighing underwater; measuring fat and lean bodyweight percentages; measuring waist girth, hip girth, and calculating waist-to-hip ratio and body mass index (BMI)/weight-to-height ratio. Fat norms are 13–25% for men, 22–32% for women; 16–20% for men, 19–20% for women are recommended; >25% for men, >35% for women constitute obesity.

## YMCA FLEXIBILITY TEST

The YMCA Flexibility Test involves initial aerobic warmup and hamstring stretching. Then the person sits on the floor, knees straight, with a yardstick or tape measure between the legs. He or she drops the head, exhales; and reaches forward, fingertips together, as far as possible and holds the position. The tester measures reach distance to the nearest ¼ in–½ in/5mm–1cm, and scores the test by the best of three trials. Adults who can reach their feet or past them are highly flexible. YMCA provides flexibility norms. For older adults, YMCA uses AAHPERD's flexibility test and norms for this population. **Muscular strength** is tested using heavy resistance, **muscular endurance** using light resistance. Isometric contractions are static; isotonic contractions use movement with constant resistance. The grip test measures hand strength. YMCA may use dynamometers, strain gauges, load cells, or cable tensiometer instruments to measure strength. Chin-ups, push-ups, sit-ups, and curl-ups are also used. Sit-ups are avoided with people having weak abdominal muscles and/or back problems. YMCA-specific tests include the 1-minute Half-Sit-Up and Bench Press Tests; online calculators are available for both.

## ASSESSMENT TOOLS FOR MEASURING SELF-EFFICACY

Included among many means of measuring self-efficacy are:

- The **Generalized Self-Efficacy (GSE) scale** (Schwarzer and Jerusalem, 1995). This instrument measures an individual's confidence for setting goals, making efforts to achieve them, and persisting in those efforts. It focuses on a person's self-efficacy in terms of optimism, coping with everyday problems and adversity, and adaptation to changes.
- The **Skill Confidence Inventory (SCI) scale** (Betz et al, 1996) is used by career counselors to measure vocational self-efficacy. It focuses on an individual's perceived confidence for succeeding at specific activities, coursework, and tasks. It contains six General Confidence Themes/GCT scales, each having 10 items. Each scale is scored by the mean/average of responses, indicating perceived confidence levels from 1/No Confidence to 5/Complete Confidence. High skill confidence corresponds to a 3.5 or higher score. Testers usually combine the SCI with the Strong Interest Inventory (SII) scale for vocational interests. Self-efficacy is characterized as domain-specific: the SCI is specific to the vocational domain; the Mathematics Self-Efficacy Scale (MSES, Betz and Hackett 1983) is specific to the mathematics domain. Scores range from 0/Not at all difficult to 9/Extremely difficult.

## AFFECTIVE ASSESSMENTS

To plan an affective survey, identify your research questions, objectives, and survey type. To develop it, identify the response format and which types of items to use; plan how to score the responses; decide which demographic information to collect and how to collect it; write the directions for responding to the survey; format the survey items; and then review and revise the instrument. Some fixed-response formats include:

- **Adjective checklists**: These are easy to write, but cannot be scored numerically except for the number of adjectives included.
- **Behavioral checklists**: These provide information about the respondents' experiences, but precisely specifying the behaviors is a challenge.
- **Ranking formats**: These assess the relative status of interests, activities, items, etc., in the respondents' perceptions/opinions, but provide no data regarding their intensity.
- **Likert-type scales**: These give numerical scores, can address numerous subjects, offer a variety of anchors, and give a range of responses; however, it can be hard to interpret scores in the middle of the range.
- **Semantic differential scales**: These also provide a range of responses and also yield detailed information regarding concepts. However, they are limited to one concept per set.

## ASSESSMENTS OF LEISURE

### FREE TIME BOREDOM ASSESSMENT

The Free Time Boredom assessment (Ragheb & Merydith, 1995) is a self-report assessment, originally developed for research uses, appropriate for respondents with normal cognitive function and written at a 4th-grade reading level. The purpose of this instrument is to establish how easily an individual becomes bored; what he or she does with free time; whether he or she has options of leisure/recreational activities sufficient for making good use of free time; whether the person's leisure activities are relevant; and whether leisure/recreational activities include physical activity. This test identifies four different aspects of boredom or leisure:

- **Meaningfulness**: Whether the person evinces purpose or focus during free time
- **Mental involvement**: Whether the individual has enough to think about during free time and finds the thoughts satisfying emotionally

- **Speed of time**: Whether the respondent has enough purposeful, satisfying activities to fill free time
- **Physical involvement**: Whether the person engages in enough physical movement during leisure time to be satisfying.

## LEISURE ATTITUDE MEASUREMENT AND IDYLL ARBOR LEISURE BATTERY

The **Leisure Attitude Measurement** (LAM; Beard & Ragheb, 1982), formerly called the Leisure Attitude Scale, originally developed for research purposes, is a self-report for cognitively high-functioning respondents to identify their attitudes regarding leisure. It identifies three areas of leisure attitudes: cognitive (beliefs, general knowledge, etc.); affective (feelings, liking and evaluations of experiences, etc.); and behavioral (past and present participation, intentions). Respondents agree or disagree with statements (e.g., that leisure participation uses their time wisely, that leisure activities are important, that people often make friends during leisure activity). It also has a Spanish version.

**The Idyll Arbor Leisure Battery** (IALB) includes a Leisure Attitude Measurement, a Leisure Motivation Scale, a Leisure Interest Measure, and a Leisure Satisfaction Measure. This battery includes an executive summary which provides examples of suitable interventions based on the scores that a client receives on each of these assessments. This instrument also includes a summary of the participant's affect (mood) and mannerisms observed during the administration of the assessments.

## LEISURESCOPE PLUS, TEEN LEISURESCOPE PLUS, AND LIFE SATISFACTION SCALE

The **Leisurescope Plus and Teen Leisurescope Plus** (Schenk, 1980s) are two assessment tools designed for assessing adult and adolescent clients respectively, both with high levels of cognitive functioning. These instruments are intended to identify areas of leisure in which the respondent has high degrees of interest and is emotionally motivated to participate and to identify individuals who need experiences providing high arousal levels. The tests utilize pictures. The manuals offer suggestions for administering them in different settings.

The **Life Satisfaction Scale** (LSS; Lohmann, 1976) informs leisure attitudes and barriers. It is a self-report, appropriate for clients with moderate to no cognitive impairment. Similar to the Philadelphia Geriatric Center's Morale Scale, it gives statements for respondents to agree/disagree with (e.g., "I feel miserable most of the time" or "I never dreamed I could be as lonely as I am now").

## STATE TECHNICAL INSTITUTE LEISURE ASSESSMENT PROCESS AND LEISURE ASSESSMENT INVENTORY

The **Leisure part of the State Technical Institute Assessment Process** (STIAP)/**State Technical Institute Leisure Assessment Process** (STILAP; Navar & Clancy) means to help adults and adolescents with physical, intellectual, psychological, or developmental disabilities attain balanced lifestyles by assessing their patterns of leisure participation, leisure skills; classifying participation patterns into areas of leisure competency; and providing guidelines for future involvement in leisure programs. This instrument extends the typical activity checklist format, including 123 activities. Respondents indicate interest (I), some (S) or much (M) interest. The test includes 14 competencies; for example, physical skills with opportunities to carry over in future years; physical skills that can be done alone; activities depending on outdoor environment, etc.

The **Leisure Assessment Inventory** (LAI; Hawkins et al, 1997), originally developed for adults and seniors with developmental disabilities, also applies for middle-aged/older adults with moderate to no cognitive disabilities and measures adults' leisure participation and behaviors. Four subscales are the Leisure Activity Participation Index, indicating involvement amount and repertoire; Leisure

Preference Index; Leisure Interest Index, showing unfulfilled activities; and Leisure Constraints, external and internal. It utilizes pictures designed for adults aged 50+ years.

## ASSESSMENT TOOLS FOR MOTIVATIONS AND INTERESTS REGARDING LEISURE ACTIVITIES

Additional assessment tools for motivations and interests regarding leisure activities include:

- The **Leisure Motivation Scale** (LMS; Beard & Ragheb, 1983), originally developed for research purposes, is appropriate for measuring motivations for leisure participation via self-reporting by clients with high cognitive functioning. Four main motivators identified are competence mastery, stimulus avoidance, social, and intellectual. Respondents indicate agreement or disagreement with statements (e.g., that expanding their interests, being with others, or learning about themselves are reasons for engaging in leisure activities).
- The **Leisure Interest Measure** (LIM; Beard & Ragheb, 1990), also a self-report for cognitively high-functioning respondents, measures interest in eight domains of leisure activities: physical, social, cultural, service, reading, artistic, mechanical, and outdoor. Statements include liking to read, to be outdoors, or to create art, etc., during one's free time. Both instruments have Spanish versions.
- The **Assessment of Leisure and Recreation Involvement** (LRI; Ragheb, 1996), a self-report for respondents with moderate/no cognitive impairment, measures perception of leisure/recreation involvement, not only participation. Six cognitive/emotional elements influencing activity participation are: interest in activity, activity importance, pleasure from activity, activity centrality to self-perception, activity absorption/intensity, and activity meaning. Respondents agree/disagree with statements about pleasure, value, and occupation from activities, etc.

## LEISURE DIAGNOSTIC BATTERY AND LEISURE SATISFACTION MEASURE

The **Leisure Diagnostic Battery** (LDB; Witt & Ellis, 1982) is probably the TR assessment instrument that has been researched most. It was originally developed to use in schools. It is self-reported and has a computerized form. It includes short forms for adolescent and adult respondents and can be administered for persons with or without disabilities. The LDB measures leisure needs, playfulness, barriers to leisure engagement, depth of leisure involvement, perceived leisure competence and control, and an inventory of leisure preferences, via several scales.

The **Leisure Satisfaction Measure** (LSM, formerly Leisure Satisfaction Scale; Beard & Ragheb, 1980) is used in assessment of cognitively high-functioning clients. It is a self-report, originally developed for research, and includes a Spanish-language version. Respondents indicate agreement/disagreement with statements like "My leisure activities are very interesting to me/help me relax/provide opportunities to try new things", etc. It aims to measure how well clients feel leisure is meeting their needs. It categorizes needs as physiological, psychological, educational, social, relaxation, and aesthetic.

## GATHERING BASELINE ASSESSMENT DATA

TRSs must collect baseline data about how a client currently functions in various domains or areas. These include **cognitive behaviors**, which influence how a client can process information and learn; **social behaviors,** which influence how a client interacts with other people, engages in community life and major life activities, and whether the client will be socially included; **physical behaviors**, which influence client physical and emotional health, movement, sensation; **self-care, leisure activity**, and prevention of secondary conditions; **psychological behaviors**, which influence client emotional wellbeing and the value the client perceives in TR/RT interventions, **client-therapist interactions**, and leisure and recreational activity; and **leisure and play**

**behaviors,** which influence client health and functioning in life and leisure and inform effective, efficient TRS service and program design by providing information on client cultural values and disabilities. To obtain assessment data, TRSs use systematic observations of the client, both obtrusively in controlled settings and unobtrusively in natural settings; client performance testing (e.g., measuring strength and balance for fall prevention); client self-report measures, like structured and unstructured client and caregiver interviews, and self-administered surveys or questionnaires; and secondary sources (e.g., family, intake records, official, and team documents).

## UTILIZING BASELINE DATA TO INFORM TRS PLANNING

During assessment, a TRS identifies the client's world view and the cultural context for the TR/RT process, and the specific liabilities, assets, and resources of the individual client related to these. The TRS must collect baseline data about the client's physical, cognitive, psychological, spiritual, and leisure functioning. This information will enable the TRS to identify the client's present status in each domain, client limitations, strengths, expectations, interests, and program needs. This baseline data and the TRS's determination of these client factors will serve as the basis for the TRS to design an individualized plan for the client. This plan will include diagnosing the client's conditions; treating them; rehabilitating the client; educating the client; and/or improving the client's health, functional abilities, and leisure wellbeing. Interventions are meant to effect functional and/or behavioral changes that will enhance leisure and quality of life from the client's perspective. The changes achieved through participating in a TR/RT program will be measured in comparison to the baselines the TRS has identified through assessment data. Baseline assessment data help TRSs decide which programs will be most effective for individual clients or client groups.

## FUNCTIONAL SKILLS ASSESSMENT

A functional skills assessment may include evaluation of the following:

- **Access in the community**: The RT must assess what resources are available in the community, qualifications and/or costs for utilization, and methods of access. For example, the RT may assess what gyms, exercise facilities, and parks are available within 5 miles of the patient's home and their costs or membership requirements if helping the patient plan an exercise program.
- **Use of social media**: The RT should assess not only the client's understanding and use of the various social media (Facebook, Twitter, Blogs, Websites) but also the type of Internet connection the client has (if any), the speed, and the cost.
- **Transportation**: The RT should assess whether the client is able to safely drive, has a license, and has a motor vehicle or must depend on others or public transportation. If dependent on public transportation, the RT should assess the nearest bus stops or stations, the costs, and any special programs (such as door-to-door service) that the transportation authority may offer to clients with disabilities.

## BEHAVIORAL OBSERVATION

Naturalistic observation, also called *behavioral* or *field observation*, is frequently used by social and behavioral scientists. It is one of the most fundamental assessment tools that they use because it enables them to observe the behavior of individuals in their natural or usual environments. The closer a setting is to the individual's home or real-life circumstances, the more the person's behaviors will reflect his or her typical behaviors when not under observation. TRSs, like other professionals practicing treatment/therapy, must accurately assess client behaviors before, during, and after treatment. Hence, they must consider how representative the observed performance is of the client's normal functioning. On the basis of naturalistic or field observations, TRSs can make evaluations of the nature of the client's needs or problem(s). They can determine which type of intervention they should provide. They can assess how the client responds to specific treatment interventions through behavioral observations. And they can ultimately evaluate how effective the program they design and implement is for meeting the client's needs. A contemporary consideration is that in the brief treatments now required, activities for client education, rehabilitation, and/or treatment often subsequently become diagnostic assessment components.

## GUIDELINES FOR BEHAVIORAL OBSERVATION

When making behavioral observations of a client/prospective client, the TRS should try to observe the person in a variety of settings that are or represent the most typical and/or frequent settings currently in the individual's life, as the person's behaviors may vary among places, times, and situations. Observations should be made systematically. If the TRS has identified specific client behaviors, the observational record should operationally and clearly describe/depict it/them. The TRS can use one, several, or all of these **procedures**:

- **Record a narrative** describing specific skills the client demonstrates; which kinds of instructions the client responds to best; types, frequency, and duration of the social interactions demonstrated; and client personal appearance.
- **Interval recording/time sampling**: record at certain time intervals, whether a behavior occurs or not. One disadvantage is using this method alone may not accurately show on an ongoing basis how often a behavior occurs.
- **Event sampling**: wait until an identified behavior occurs, and then record its duration and frequency. One disadvantage with this method alone is if the client never demonstrates the behavior.
- **Rating scales**, which offer more structured techniques for observation and recording.

## ABC DATA COLLECTION IN BEHAVIORAL OBSERVATION

ABC in the context of data collection stands for **antecedent, behavior, and consequences**. According to behaviorist principles, an antecedent is some event that occurs prior to a behavior and serves as a stimulus that elicits a certain response from an individual. That response is a behavior. After the individual demonstrates that behavior, which must be outwardly observable, there is some consequence occurring as a result of the behavior. That consequence may be reinforcing, increasing the probability he or she will repeat the behavior, or punishing, decreasing the probability of behavior repetition. Consequences can include no response from people or the environment. However, if the behavior was intended to get attention, no response does have an effect on the individual by not providing that reinforcement, making the individual (eventually) less likely to repeat the behavior; this is called extinction. The original behaviorist acronyms were, first, S-R, stimulus-response; then modified to S-O-R, stimulus-organism-response to include the individual responding to the stimulus. After behavior modification techniques progressed, the acronym ABC became popular, especially in educational and healthcare settings. S-O-R and ABC have essentially the same meaning.

When anyone, including a TRS, uses the ABC data collection method, he or she can discover why an individual performs a given behavior. This is part of a **functional behavior analysis.** All behaviors have a function: to get something (objects, nourishment, rest, attention, gratification, stimulation, help, relief, control, power, etc.) or get away from something (escape). According to behaviorist principles, if we want to change a behavior, we must first determine why the individual demonstrates it. It is not effective simply to punish a behavior every time it happens. First, punishment is not as powerful as reinforcement. Second, it is impossible to present consequences every single time a behavior occurs: the practitioner will not always be in the individual's presence. Third, punishment tends to be associated with the person presenting it and the setting; its effects often do not transfer to other settings/situations and people. Since punishment has limited usefulness, it is more effective to reinforce an incompatible or more acceptable behavior that achieves the same function.

### USING BEHAVIORAL OBSERVATIONS TO INFORM SUBSEQUENT TREATMENT PLANNING

Suppose a TRS is conducting comprehensive assessment of a new client referred for rehabilitation following injury. This client could not walk due to non–weight-bearing foot and ankle fractures. Now the bones have healed; the orthopedic physician/surgeon confirmed she can bear weight again. Due to substantial soft tissue injuries, a history of repeated injuries to the same extremity, and several months being nonambulatory, the orthopedist ordered physical therapy (PT). The PT also recommended TR/RT. Also consider this client indicated during an intake interview that even before the injury, she was quite sedentary and preferred sitting and watching TV/reading. During assessment, the TRS could use behavioral observation to measure when/how often the client stands up/walks in typical settings and situations and record reasons for standing/walking. Functional behavior analysis will inform the TRS's treatment plans. The TRS can select activities that motivate the client and reinforcers (rewards) the client values for becoming more physically active, to support restoring ambulation skills.

### BEHAVIORAL OBSERVATIONS IN THE CLIENT'S NATURAL ENVIRONMENT

TR/RT services and programs frequently take place in settings with which the clients are familiar. As a result, TRSs are often able to observe and record behaviors that their clients do not display while staying in hospitals or clinics on an inpatient basis or while in the presence of other therapists. As one example, observing a client navigate through an obstacle course in a hospital that the TRS has designed will not yield as accurate an assessment of a client's capacity for independently maintaining ambulation as observing the client during outings in the community and how well the client masters navigation in relation to natural environmental accessibility barriers. When the TRS records these kinds of observations in the client's individual program plan (IPP) and discusses them with other care providers during meetings and conferences, providing this information helps to assure that everybody who interacts with the client will consistently respond to support the client's strengths, needs, and goals.

### COGNITIVE BEHAVIORAL ASSESSMENT

Thinking processes regulate body movements and the behavioral aspects of participating in TR/RT, so they are important for TRSs to assess. Cognition affects strategic decisions during board, table, and card games; choices of experiences among alternatives; and capacity for processing information and learning in leisure, recreation, and life. Cognitive functioning involves a series of processes. At their simplest, these are concrete behaviors. They progressively become more complex, with more behaviors and increasingly abstract thinking involved. For example, recalling lists of items/facts/rules is less challenging than producing original artworks. According to Bloom's Taxonomy (1956), the hierarchy of cognitive difficulty from lowest to highest is knowledge/recall, comprehension, application, analysis, synthesis, and evaluation. Evaluating situations and deciding on actions appropriate to situations represent the highest cognitive difficulty level. Choosing alternative travel options and managing money, as often required in inclusion activities, are at this level. When assessing cognitive behaviors, TRSs test areas including orientation to place, time, and person; arousal, selective attention, alternating attention, concentration; recognition; short-term, long-term, and retrieval memory; language; sequencing; counting; calculation; decision-making; problem-solving; planning; organization; and abstraction.

## SOCIAL BEHAVIOR ASSESSMENT

Since many other professions disregard social skills, which are important to wellbeing, TRS social assessment is critical. Social functioning includes attitudes, behaviors, and language individuals exhibit in relationships, during interactions, and participation in work, volunteer, and formal and informal recreation experiences. Social interaction is both a primary leisure experience and a result of leisure activity motivating participation in other leisure/life experiences. Because social competence is multifaceted, people with inadequate social skills need direct instruction for future success and risk reduction. The progressive hierarchy of social behaviors is intra-individual or solitary (such as daydreaming), extra-individual (such as playing Solitaire), aggregate interaction (parallel but not interactive participation in activities in the same environment), inter-individual interaction (such as 1:1 competition), unilateral interaction (a team of individuals competing against one individual), multilateral interaction (individuals in a group competing equally), intragroup interaction (such as two or more individuals collaborating on a project), and intergroup interaction (two or more groups competing against each other). TRSs assess social behaviors including communication, same-sex and opposite-sex interactions, cooperation, sportsman-ship, peer/other-age relations, sharing, taking turns, and waiting. Instrumental skills involve getting information/getting/keeping jobs; affiliation skills involve sharing feelings. Influences by and on social skills/deficits are reciprocal with other domains.

## PHYSICAL BEHAVIOR ASSESSMENT

TRSs assess physical behaviors including gross and fine motor skills, sensory utilization, perception, mobility, balance, coordination, flexibility, strength, and endurance. Physical skills are important for performing self-care, preventing secondary conditions, maintaining physical and emotional health, and participating in active leisure lifestyles. While some physical abilities are required for most leisure experiences, some need fewer or more; for example, swimming and running require more physical skills than painting and acting. Physical behavior assessments measure the number of body parts used and the frequency, intensity, and duration of each activity. The more each of these increases, the more difficult the physical activity becomes. Physical behavior assessments enable TRSs to evaluate a client's current functioning levels and residual abilities (functions unaffected by disability) for specific skills like responding to sensations, grasping and releasing, and ambulating. TRSs often collaborate with PTs, OTs, SLPs, and audiologists to adapt assessments to prevent clients' sensation and wellbeing levels from compromising their performance.

## PSYCHOLOGICAL BEHAVIOR ASSESSMENT

When TRSs assess a client's psychological behaviors, they are concerned with how the client communicates or expresses emotions. When assessing psychological behaviors, a TRS would evaluate the client's emotional stability; attitudes toward self; expression; locus of control; anger control and management; and what value the client assigns to the satisfaction he or she gets from various friendship, leisure, and other interactions and experiences as measures of the person's emotional status. A hierarchy of psychological behaviors, from least to most demanding or emotionally involving (Krathwohl et al, 1964), is receiving (listening to others), responding (demonstrating interest), valuing; organization (demonstrating responsibility for one's own behaviors), and characterization (showing consistent patterns of behavior). TR/RT intervention can improve the client's appropriate expression of satisfaction, enjoyment, and other feelings and stress management. Measures of a client's emotional wellbeing include the value he or she accords to interactions with the TRS during interventions and to leisure in general.

## SPIRITUALITY ASSESSMENT

Subjective wellbeing is influenced by spirituality as an integrative health measure. Spirituality involves feeling connected to self, nature, and a higher power; gives life meaning; and influences individual health perceptions. Research shows the impact of spirituality on healing and wellbeing. Spirituality can be related to meditation, relaxation, art, music, wilderness experiences, relationships, nonverbal communication, and other experiences evoking physical and mental peace. In services to aging adults, spiritual needs include feeling competent, successful, useful, and connected. In hospice, palliative care includes addressing spiritual health. TRSs subjectively assess optimism, hope for the future, and purpose/meaning in life informing decision-making and relationships. They observe commitment to personal fulfillment, ethical responses, and motivational levels. Many leisure wellness assessments include spiritual health items. In spiritual assessments, TRSs identify isolation, anger, etc., causing spiritual isolation, and nature, pets, relationships, humor, and other strategies promoting meaning and comfort. Assessing leisure and play behaviors indicates overall health and life abilities and functioning, provides baseline data for planning and evaluating TR/RT interventions, and assures compliance with professional practice standards and accrediting associations' care standards. Assessing leisure knowledge, interests, needs, barriers, assets, and patterns helps TRSs design services/programs that consider client values and lifestyles.

## PATIENT INTERVIEW
### PROBLEM IDENTIFICATION

Although assessment is regarded as the initial phase of the APIE (Assessment, Planning, Implementation, and Evaluation) process, clinical authorities also point out that even after the initial assessment is completed, it is best to view assessment as an ongoing process because changes will occur during intervention, so additional assessments will be necessary. Some questions that a TRS can ask a client during an initial interview to assist with identifying the client's presenting problem include the following:

- Ask the client what has brought him or her to the TRS today. Or ask what the main problem is for which the client is seeing the TRS.
- Ask how long this problem has existed, or how long the condition/injury/illness/disability has been a problem.
- Ask whether the client has noticed times and/or places in which the problem is not as bad, and seems worse.
- Ask if anything like the current problem/situation ever occurred before. If the client says yes, ask how this happened and how he or she tried to resolve the problem last time it happened.
- Ask how often the client has experienced this problem. Also ask who is affected by/involved in the current situation/problem.

### ASCERTAINING CLIENT GOALS

When interviewing a new client, the TRS will first want to identify the client's presenting problem. Then he or she should ask the client what his or her goals are for TR/RT. Some examples of questions the TRS can ask the client include the following:

- What is your goal(s) for participating in TR/RT?
- What would you like to get out of this appointment?
- What changes would you like to happen for you?
- What things would you like to be able to do that you cannot do right now?

- What are some circumstances now that you want to remain the same?
- How will you know that you will not have to come back here anymore?
- Regarding symptoms, the TRS can ask the client whether he or she has recently lost or gained weight; whether he or she has recently noticed any changes in sleeping, eating, concentration, or mood; how much he or she uses alcohol and other drugs; and how much the current problem has affected his or her health and ability to perform home, school, or work duties.

## LISTENING TECHNIQUES DURING THE CLIENT INTERVIEW

Listening is an important element in the client interview. **Passive listening**, which entails not interrupting clients and accepting silent periods, is necessary at times. **Active listening** involves restating the client's communications for confirmation or denial and correction; reflecting how the client seems to feel; and putting oneself in the client's place. Some pitfalls include being too eager to help to listen adequately; being ignorant of cultural attitude and communication differences; being fatigued; being near burnout; judging what the client says as right or wrong, based on one's own cultural biases and/or personal perspectives; and responding not to client context, experiences, and feelings, but to client diagnosis. New TRSs may depend initially on knowledge from courses and books for listening behaviors until they gain enough experience to be able to recognize each client's uniqueness. New TRSs may also respond not to the person's feelings or context but to the factual content of what clients say. Even autistic or mentally ill clients whose speech presents as obsessed with facts still convey themes hidden in their messages, which TRSs must help them clarify and should then reflect to them. Another danger is sympathizing instead of empathizing: feeling sorry for a client's plight can cause subjectivity and bias.

## ADDITIONAL CONSIDERATIONS FOR CLIENT INTERVIEWS

When interviewing children and others with limited attention spans, keep interviews brief. Adjust your language to fit the client's educational level, social class, ethnicity, age, etc. When listening to a client's responses to questions, especially open-ended questions that can evoke lengthy responses, listen selectively and focus on themes you notice running through the client's communication. Listen to paragraphs rather than sentences, phrases, or words. When responding, use "I" statements to take ownership/responsibility for your own feelings; encourage the client to follow suit. Before giving a client feedback on his or her messages, mentally summarize what you think you heard the client say. When offering feedback, use the same level of vocabulary that the client uses. Before continuing, speak directly to the client and clarify any statements that may have been overly vague or generalized. Use timing to avoid interrupting the client with your responses; respond at times that facilitate the client's communication. Avoid focusing on culturally sensitive subjects or emotionally charged words; instead, listen to the client from a contextual perspective.

## STRUCTURED VS. UNSTRUCTURED INTERVIEWS

Structured interviews are formal interviews with predetermined questions, similar to job interviews. Questions are standardized across clients, asked in consistent order, not flexible to changes/additions, and closed-ended. Rather than "Tell me about..." questions, they tend to require yes/no responses; specific information like how much/how often/how long/what/where/when/who/why; and shorter responses like words/phrases. Some advantages include closed questions in fixed sets, making them easy to quantify and replicate, thus to test for reliability, and quick administration for the maximum number of interviews in a short time. Disadvantages include inflexibility, requiring following the interview schedule, prohibiting impromptu new questions. Also, responses are quantitative and lack detail: interviewers obtain little insight into motivations.

Unstructured or **"discovery" interviews** are like guided conversations. Questions are open-ended, can be asked in any order, and may be removed or added. Advantages include flexibility: questions can be changed according to individual responses. They evoke qualitative data, enabling respondents to choose their words and speak in depth, facilitating interviewer understanding. Disadvantages include taking more time, both to interview and interpret information, and more time and expense for training in interviewing skills.

## ASSESSING VISUAL ACUITY

Visual acuity is measured as the number of feet at which someone can read a number of lines of printed characters on a Snellen eye chart, compared to the number of feet at which someone with normal vision can read them. This comparison is expressed as a ratio: 20/20 or normal vision means someone can read the number of lines on the chart that people can normally read at 20 feet. Someone who sees at 20 feet what normal eyes see at 200 feet has 20/200 vision.

- 20/200 in the better eye after correction is defined as **legally blind.**
- 20/200 to 20/70 in the better eye after correction, or a 30° or lower visual field, is **low vision.**
- A 20° or lower field of vision is **tunnel vision.**
- Vision measured at 5/200 to 10/200 is **travel vision**.
- 3/200 to 5/200—usually moving, not still, objects—is **motion perception.**
- Vision below 3/200—seeing bright light from 3 feet away but not detecting movement—is **light perception.**
- Inability to see strong light shined into the eye is **total blindness.**
- Those born blind have **congenital blindness;** losing eyesight after birth is **adventitious blindness.**

### REFRACTIVE ERRORS, MUSCULAR IMBALANCES, GENETIC CONDITIONS, AND INJURIES

Vision impairments include refractive errors, muscular imbalances, genetic disorders, and injury-induced impairments:

- **Refractive errors**: *Myopia*: nearsightedness, being able to see clearly near but not far. *Hyperopia*: farsightedness, being able to see clearly far but not near. *Astigmatism*: blurred near and far vision. *Presbyopia*: aging-related farsightedness (loss of focus). *Bifocal vision*: nearsighted people also develop presbyopia.
- **Muscular imbalances**: *Nystagmus*: rapid vertical and horizontal eye movements. *Strabismus*: crossed or "wall"/turned-out eyes. *Amblyopia*/"lazy eye": impaired binocular focusing, making one eye dominant and the other weak.
- **Genetic disorders/hereditary conditions**: *Achromatic vision*: color-blindness—total, or red-green. *Albinism*: lack of pigmentation causes visual refractive errors, photosensitivity, and other problems. *Retinitis pigmentosa*: the eyes' rods and cones fail to regenerate, causing tunnel vision/central vision loss and night-blindness. *Cataracts*: congenital or aging-related cloudiness/opacity on eye lenses, causing impaired vision and blindness if not removed. *Conjunctivitis:* inflammation of conjunctiva/inner eyelid lining and scleral covering. *Diabetic retinopathy:* retinal hemorrhages from vascular changes cause blindness. *Glaucoma:* increased inner-eye fluid pressure impairs eyesight, beginning with peripheral vision.
- **Injuries/accidents**: Detached retina(s); dislocated retina(s); punctured eyeballs; and retinopathy of prematurity (ROP) in infants, caused by inadequate incubator oxygen regulation.

## HEARING ASSESSMENT

Audiological assessment and measurements include the following:

- Sound loudness is **intensity**, measured in decibels (dB). 0 dB can be heard barely/about 50% of the time with normal hearing; >100 dB causes pain.
- **Frequency** determines high/medium/low sound pitches measured in Hertz (Hz). Humans normally hear 20–20,000 Hz.
- **Spectrum**, from single-frequency pure tones to complex speech/musical tones, determines sound *timbre*.
- Aging-related hearing loss/**presbycusis** begins with loss of high-frequency sounds, impairing *discrimination* of consonant sounds, especially unvoiced (/s/, /t/, /p/, /f/, /ʃ/, /tʃ/, /θ/).
- Hearing of 26–40 dB at all tested frequencies represents **mild hearing loss:** one cannot understand whispered speech. 41–55 dB represents **moderate hearing loss:** one can understand conversation at normal loudness from 3–5 feet, but not farther. 56–70 dB represents **moderately severe hearing loss**: one can understand only loud speech at close ranges. 71–90 dB represents **severe hearing loss**: one may hear loud voices around a foot away from the ear(s). 91 dB or higher represents **profound hearing loss**: one can sense vibrations, but not tonal patterns.
- **Hard of hearing** people have hearing loss but can process spoken language with/without hearing aids.
- **Deaf** people cannot process spoken language with/without hearing aids.

### CONDUCTIVE VS. SENSORINEURAL HEARING LOSS

**Conductive hearing losses** are caused by physical obstructions in the conduction of sound waves from the outer or middle ear to the inner ear. For example, wax buildups in the ear canal; middle ear infections (*otitis media*) causing fluid, pus, and scar tissue in the middle ear; or *otosclerosis,* immobilizing the ossicles (tiny bones) in the middle ear that conduct sound, can cause conductive hearing losses. Conductive hearing losses are often curable, reversible, or treatable. People with conductive hearing losses generally benefit more from hearing aids than those with sensorineural deafness.

**Sensorineural hearing losses** are caused by damage to/defects in the hair cells (*cilia*) inside the inner ear's cochlea, and/or the auditory and/or acoustic nerves that convert sound waves into acoustic energy and carry the nerve impulses from the cochlea to the brain. Sensorineural hearing loss can be caused by congenital defects; damage in utero, during, or after birth; infections; contagious diseases; aging; or long-term exposure to very loud sounds. Unlike conductive hearing losses, sensorineural hearing losses are irreversible. For people whose cochleas/cochlear nerve cells were destroyed or never developed, cochlear implants combined with hearing aids and aural rehabilitation/habilitation training can restore/provide some hearing.

### DUAL SENSORY IMPAIRMENTS

An individual who has vision measured at 20/200 can see at 20 feet what he or she should be able to see at 200 feet, or has a field of vision of 20° or less, and also has a hearing loss of 25 dB or more, is defined as having a **dual-sensory impairment**. Assessing and treating these impairments has additional considerations because one sense cannot be used to compensate for deficits in the other as easily. These individuals will need additional input via other senses, with greater information amounts and redundancy, to respond to assessment and treatment. People with some conductive hearing loss—loss of air and bone conduction from the outer or middle ear to the inner ear—combined with some sensorineural hearing loss—loss of nerve conduction from inner ear to brain—have mixed hearing loss. **Mixed hearing losses** are more common among elderly people. Whereas sensorineural hearing losses associated with aging are typically worst at higher frequencies, **hearing loss from exposure to very loud noises** typically causes a precipitous hearing loss at middle frequency, around 4,000 Hz, with lower and higher frequencies unaffected.

## ASSESSING MEMORY

A TRS must determine how a client retains and retrieves information to assess how he can learn during therapy. Some clients with brain injuries remember past experiences but cannot retain new information. Others have both types of **memory loss**. Some have retrograde amnesia, meaning they cannot remember events before injury, but may be able to acquire new memories. Some clients with intellectual disability have difficulty remembering instructions/information without extensive, consistent repetition.

- **Short-term memory** involves temporary storage of small amounts of information, as in rehearsal (e.g., repeating phone numbers until dialing).
- **Working memory** refers to processes not only for temporarily storing information (short-term memory), but also organizing and manipulating it.
- Attending to the information enables its transition into **long-term memory,** which can last days to many decades, though it can eventually be forgotten. Popular standardized IQ tests assess digit span (repeating series of numbers, including reversing them) and verbal memory (e.g., repeating series of words).
- **Explicit/declarative memory** is conscious long-term memory, including *semantic* memory about the world and *episodic memory* about specific events.
- **Implicit/procedural memory** retains body movement and object manipulation routines, like riding bicycles, driving cars, using computers, etc., which can be important in TR/RT.

## ASSESSING PROBLEM SOLVING SKILLS

Clients use problem-solving in leisure education, stress management and social skills training. Physical medicine, mental health, and rehabilitation services often use problem-solving experiences (e.g., how to gain access by negotiating physical barriers, or considering the consequences of choices). Problem-solving components include gathering information to identify and evaluate a problem, generating alternatives, choosing solutions, implementing solution strategies, and evaluating strategies' efficacy. In leisure experiences, clients need problem-solving and decision-making skills for self-determination. They also need them to cope with stress caused by disabilities/health conditions. Careless/impulsive problem-solving correlates with more depression symptoms; proactive problem-solving increases perceived self-control and competence. Clients with pain, strokes, spinal cord injuries, intellectual disabilities, and mental health problems, and their caregivers, benefit from problem-solving training. Some problem-solving items to assess include: identifying a problem, studying its scope, viewing a problem in multiple ways, determining a topic, asking a fundamental question, using tools to identify solution alternatives, considering the consequences of an unsolved problem, evaluating alternative solutions, establishing solution evaluation criteria, selecting the best solution, forming compromise solutions, communicating the problem-solving process to others, and applying the problem-solving process to new problems.

## ASSESSING ATTENTION SPAN

When conducting a comprehensive assessment, a TRS must include assessment of cognitive behaviors. One of these is attention span. The client's attention span can influence the assessment of the other cognitive behaviors to be assessed, because attention is a fundamental skill; if the client is unable to pay attention for long enough to the assessment items or process, the TRS will be unable to complete the assessment and obtain the data needed for establishing baseline levels and planning services. Therefore, clinicians often assess attention span before testing the other cognitive behaviors. The results of testing the attention span will also influence the TRS's planning of services/programs. Intervention for clients with head injuries or AD/HD and short attention spans could include training for gradually increasing the duration they can attend to an activity. Interventions with young children and clients with intellectual disabilities are informed by measuring their attention spans to keep activity durations appropriate. Assessment includes distractibility, thought completion, thinking/problem-solving, subtracting backward by number intervals, spelling words forward and backward, and repeating numbers forward and reversed.

## ASSESSING ORIENTATION

Orientation refers to whether an individual is aware of basic aspects of reality or not. The standard types of orientation assessed during mental status examinations are orientation to place, orientation to time, and orientation to person. Someone oriented to all three may or may not necessarily be mentally healthy otherwise, but can be confirmed as not delirious or significantly demented. For example, people suffering brain injuries; alcohol, drug, or other substance intoxication, abuse, and/or withdrawal symptoms; or Alzheimer's disease may not be oriented. People with severe intellectual disabilities may not demonstrate all three types of orientation. Disorientation can be temporary, as with substance intoxication/withdrawal; or persistent/chronic, as in Alzheimer's disease. To determine orientation to time, assessors ask what season it is, what day of the week, today's month, date, and year, and what time it is. Orientation to place involves asking if clients know where they are, where they live, where they work, etc. Orientation to person includes individuals' names, how old they are, and to identify family members, close friends, or others present whom they know well.

## ASSESSING SAFETY AWARENESS

TRSs must identify safety awareness presence and levels before planning/implementing therapy to know how much supervision vs. independence clients will initially require during activities. For example, brain-injured/demented/intellectually disabled clients may not be able to judge safe air or water temperatures, avoid burns, choose appropriate clothing, judge safe ambulation distances, know when/how to talk to/not talk to strangers, avoid medication overdoses, remember to take medications on schedule, ambulate on foot/in wheelchairs safely on ice/wet surfaces, etc. Safety awareness skills interact with problem-solving skills and reasoning abilities. Safety awareness is a vital skill set not only during RT/TR interventions, home and community leisure and recreational activities, but also at home, with security measures; in bedrooms and bathrooms; in kitchens, with water, appliances, cleaning products, etc.; using wheelchairs/assistive devices; with diet and swallowing; with health behaviors and medications; on floors and stairs; in the community, indoors and outdoors; and for general safety precautions. The Source for Safety (Fogle, Reece, & White, 2008) is the first cognitively-oriented tool for both assessing and training safety awareness. Scores and difficulty levels are correlated with the FIM, MDS, and ASHA Functional Communication Measures.

## ASSESSING SOCIAL SKILLS

The TRS needs to assess an individual's social skills for interacting with other people. Not only does the TRS need to determine what kinds of interactions the client will initially be able to tolerate and know how to engage in during therapy, he or she also needs to know what skills the client has, lacks, and/or needs for interacting socially with others following treatment, to enable community reintegration, facilitate leisure and recreational activities at home and in the community after intervention, to prevent social isolation following treatment, and to enable general success in life. The TRS will assess how the client behaves in groups, initiates and maintains 1:1 and group conversations, participates in activities, both passively and actively; how the client competes and cooperates with others; the clients' ability to negotiate, share, and empathize with others; the client's perceptions and demonstrations of personal boundaries and space; how the client handles physical proximity and contact; the client's social engagement, manners, and etiquette; client issues with trust and mistrust; teamwork; sportsmanship; interaction style; and social support networks.

## ASSESSING COMMUNICATION SKILLS

### VERBAL COMMUNICATION

Communication skills include verbal and nonverbal communication. Verbal communication includes receptive and expressive skills. Receptive verbal skills involve understanding what others say and being able to read printed/written language. Expressive verbal skills involve being able to use spoken language to communicate needs, wants, feelings, thoughts, ideas, and interact socially with others. It is typical for receptive verbal skills to develop sooner and be more advanced than expressive verbal skills. Hence, children and developmentally disabled people tend to have better ability to understand what they hear than ability to express what they feel or think and tend to read better than to write at given ages or developmental stages/levels. Thus, assessors should not assume from an individual's expressive level that his or her receptive level is the same. Some verbal assessments are entirely receptive; for example, the Peabody Picture Vocabulary Test (PPVT) requires respondents only to point to pictures to match words the tester says. This is useful for assessing cognitive levels without requiring speaking or writing skills.

### NONVERBAL COMMUNICATION

Despite our society's strongly verbal orientation, nonverbal communication is equally important. In fact, research has found more than half our total communication can be nonverbal. Nonverbal communication includes eye contact, facial expressions, posture, body movements, physical gestures, haptics (touch), proxemics (personal and social physical space and distance), and vocal tones. These all interact with verbal communication. The roles nonverbal communication cues play relative to verbal messages include repeating (e.g., saying "I don't know" and then shrugging), accentuating (e.g., pounding a table to emphasize a point), contradicting (e.g., a facial expression the opposite of one's words, as in sarcasm), substituting (e.g., using one's eyes or face to communicate a message more vividly than words can), or complementing (e.g., patting someone on the back while verbally praising). Mismatched verbal vs. nonverbal communications cause mistrust, confusion, and tension. Some clients with autism spectrum disorders, intellectual disabilities, developmental delays/disabilities, voice/speech/language disorders, including physical disabilities, etc., are nonverbal, deaf/hearing-impaired, or non-English-speaking. Nonverbal assessment instruments like the Leiter International Performance Scale, Raven's Progressive Matrices, and Universal Nonverbal Intelligence Test (UNIT) are available to test their intelligence and understanding.

## ASSESSING CLIENT RELATIONSHIPS

The **Relational Assessment Questionnaire** (RAQ; Snell, 1996) is a self-report survey assessment whereby assessors can discover how people feel and think about their intimate or close relationships. Respondents rate each statement offered according to a Likert-type scale as very, moderately, somewhat, slightly, or not at all characteristic of them. Examples of statements include "I am a good partner...", "I am depressed about [my] relationship...", "I feel good about myself as a...partner", "I cannot...be happy in intimate relationships", "I'm constantly thinking about being in an intimate relationship", "I hardly ever fantasize about highly intimate relationships", "I sometimes doubt my ability to maintain a close relationship", "I feel sad when I think about my intimate experiences", etc. On the final item of 31, the respondent identifies whether the responses were based upon a current, past, or imagined intimate relationship. In the scoring instructions, author Snell identifies three scales: Relational Esteem, Relational Depression, and Relational

Preoccupation, and lists the numbers of the items that fall into each scale's category. Certain items are coded (R), indicating their responses are to be scored in the reverse order of the others.

## Skills for Establishing and Maintaining Relationships

An individual's skills for establishing and maintaining relationships are complex and involve interactions among various influencing factors. These include an individual's personality traits (extraversion, agreeableness, conscientiousness, neuroticism, and openness), individual emotional and other intelligences, the person's prior life experiences, characteristics of the particular situation, cognitive and perceptual filters, the relationship-building skills and basic communication skills the individual utilizes in the situation, the individual's outcomes, the group's outcomes, productivity, success, and consumer satisfaction. These authors define interpersonal skills as "goal-directed behaviors, including communication and relationship-building competencies, employed in interpersonal interaction episodes characterized by complex perceptual and cognitive processes, dynamic verbal and nonverbal interaction exchanges, diverse roles, motivations, and expectancies." They find effective interpersonal behavior demands different types of competence, acquired through instinct, experience, and learning concerning specific social contexts. The assessment implication is that measurements must be made in realistic settings to enable analyzing cognitive processes, attitudes, and behaviors comprising social skills.

## Assessing Gross Motor Skills

Gross motor skills involve large muscle movements like sitting, standing, walking, running, jumping, kicking, and large arm movements like throwing and catching. One way to assess gross motor skills is by using range of motion. For example, ask the client to hold an arm out and move it in a complete circle while it is fully extended. Ask the client to stand and extend one leg. Then ask the client to move the leg back and forth, left to right, and up and down. Pay attention to whether the client shows any difficulty or pain in performing these movements and/or performs them abnormally. Another way to assess gross motor skills is through game activities. Ask the client to kick a ball to test leg movement. Have the client jump rope, which allows assessment of both arm and leg movements, as well as interlimb coordination. Walking on a balance beam, playing hopscotch, and playing basketball are also good activities for assessing gross motor skills. TRSs should look for eye-hand coordination and balance difficulties and whether movements are fluid or jerky.

## Assessing Fine Motor Skills

Fine motor skills involve small muscle movements of the hands and feet, including object manipulation, which are important to many daily living activities and work skills. Some tests include asking a client to attach a clothespin to a box edge, string large beads on a shoelace, use a stapler, put a paperclip on a piece of paper, and pick up an object from the floor using only the toes. Observe performance ease/difficulty and movement smoothness. Everyday household items can be used to test object manipulation fine motor skills: ask the client to unscrew a jar lid and screw it back on; put blocks, coins, etc., into buckets/bowls/cups; use scissors to cut a straight line marked on paper; pick up and grasp differently-sized pens/pencils; and trace drawings on tracing paper. Observe difficulties/problems and task completion. Fine motor skills can also be assessed with dressing tasks: ask the client to put on a shirt and button it, put on pants and zip and snap them, and put on laced shoes and tie them. Observe task performance for abnormal movements, difficulties, and ability to complete each task independently (unassisted).

## CARDIOVASCULAR ASSESSMENT

### AEROBIC ENDURANCE TESTS

Some aerobic endurance tests involve having people exercise continuously to exhaustion (until they can no longer perform the exercise). These include the PACER Test, Aero Test, and Multistage Shuttle Run test; the $VO_2$max or maximum oxygen consumption test; a simplified form of the $VO_2$max measure called the Vmax test; the Bruce Protocol Test; the Balke Treadmill Test, which has the client walk on a treadmill until exhaustion; the University of Montreal Track Test, which is the original "beep" test to employ beep signals; and the Birtwell 40-meter Shuttle Run. Intermittent tests include rest/recovery periods and are used to test an individual's ability for playing rugby, soccer, and other sports with interval or intermittent activity that require both endurance running and brief, high-intensity sprints as well as agility, speed, and strength. Intermittent tests include Yo-Yo tests; the J.A.M. test; Soccer FIT Interval Test; FIFA Interval Test 2; and 30–15 Intermittent Shuttle Run Fitness Test.

While some aerobic fitness/endurance tests involve either exercising until exhaustion or exercising intermittently with rest periods, other tests involve **walking and/or running**. These include various tests that specify set distances or times in general. Specific walking/running aerobic endurance tests include the Miller 20m Run, 1-mile Endurance Run/Walk, Half-Mile Walk, IPFT 1km/1000m Run, 1-mile Rockport Walk Test, 1-Mile Walk Test, 1.6km/1-mile Run, PRT 1.5-mile Run, 2km Walk Test, 2.4km Run Test, APFT 2-Mile Run, PFT 3-mile Run, 3km Run, 5km Run, 6-minute Run, 6-minute Walk Test, 12-minute Cooper Test, and 15-minute Balke Test. Other tests are group-specific/sport-specific, including the 10m Beep Test for children with cerebral palsy, 10m Incremental Shuttle Walk Test for people with chronic obstructive pulmonary disease (COPD), 2km Rowing Ergometer Test, Shuttle Swim Test for water polo players, Swimming Beep Test, Critical Swim Speed Test, Swimming Step Test, 1km Swim Time Trial for triathletes, Elliptical Trainer Test, 450-yd/500m Swimming Test, Multistage Field Test for wheelchair users, 12-minute Wheelchair Aerobic Test, Ice Hockey Beep Test, Water Polo Intermittent Shuttle Test, and Loughborough Intermittent Shuttle Test for soccer players.

## AFFECTIVE ASSESSMENT

The **affective domain** is considered most challenging to assess due to its complexity and the resultant difficulty of evaluating it. It typically overlaps with the other domains. Affective assessment also offers extremely rich data since it evaluates behaviors related to feelings, attitudes, and beliefs. Two major categories of affective (and other) assessments include:

- **Records**, which provide factual descriptions of relevant incidents and behaviors and represent systematic ways of collecting data.
- **Observations**, which can be informal or formal and can be used to assess individual or group behaviors.

Some guidelines for assessment of affective behaviors include: identify behaviors or traits in advance; independently rate specific behaviors or aspects; employ suitable rating scales. Scales should include enough choices to discriminate among specific behaviors. If some items are more important, weight these as warranted. Treat assessment results/information confidentially. When assessing affective learning: first write performance objectives/criteria; identify the specific behaviors involved; confine a record or observation to 1–2 behaviors. Choose, adapt, or create instruments according to assessment needs. Determine whom to survey/observe and when. Procure as many responses/observations as possible. Identify and analyze behavioral change patterns.

## FIVE AREAS OF THE AFFECTIVE DOMAIN

The five areas of the affective domain are as follows:

- **Receiving** is characterized by demonstrating awareness; being aware of differences and characteristics; paying attention to others and their behaviors; perceiving others' characteristics and qualities; acknowledging, tolerating, and accepting differences. Interest inventories wherein respondents identify whether they like/dislike/neither like nor dislike items listed are suitable for assessment.
- **Responding** involves acting/doing, typified by showing interest in activities, cooperating with others, complying with rules, obeying guidelines, caring for others, accepting responsibility, volunteering for activities, and agreeing to try new activities. Frequency inventories in which respondents select how often do items listed are appropriate for assessment.
- **Valuing/developing attitudes** is characterized by expressing oneself; demonstrating concern; initiating plans; taking responsibility; and seeking, selecting, adopting, and utilizing resources. To assess this area, 5-point Likert-type scales ask respondents whether they strongly agree/agree/are undecided/disagree/strongly disagree with statements offered.
- **Organization** involves clarifying/explaining/arranging personal values: disclosing information about them, adapting/adjusting self and lifestyle to them, and ranking them. Open-ended questionnaires and interviews assess this area.
- **Characterization by values**, involving philosophy of life/code of conduct, is typified by influencing others; demonstrating devotion; exemplifying/ modeling; advocating; maintaining, displaying, and acting on values; supporting; and serving. Suggesting and observing appropriate actions can assess this.

## PRIMARY VS. SECONDARY DATA SOURCES

Primary sources of assessment data are obtained directly from the client. For example, when a TRS administers performance testing measures and self-reporting measures to the client and scores client responses; unobtrusively observes client behaviors in a naturalistic setting; and/or obtrusively observes client behaviors in a controlled setting, these are primary data sources. When the TRS reads the client's medical and educational records, other test results, progress notes, social histories; participates in team meetings; conducts home visits; and has informal conversations with other professionals, family members, friends and support system members, these are secondary data sources.

Secondary-source data supplements primary-source data, especially when client status (e.g., intellectual disability, communication disabilities, age) limit collecting data directly from the client. Observable facts conforming with agency protocols are objective data, uninfluenced by personal ideas, beliefs, prejudices, or emotions. Impressions, observations, and discussions from meetings/documents influenced, even biased, by personal interpretations, are subjective data. A holistic view of the client and client perceptions of health and quality of life require both objective and subjective data.

## GATHERING SECONDARY DATA

### ADDITIONAL FACTORS TO ASSESS AS SECONDARY DATA

In addition to comprehensive testing of the client, a TRS must conduct other assessments of all factors that have effects on the client, the agency where the TRS is employed and/or which is providing services to the client, and the program in which the client is or will be involved. Indicators of structure that the TRS will need to assess include the resources available from the organization(s) involved; the policies and strategic plans and statements of the departments involved; the facility in which the client will be or is being treated; the equipment available in or to the facility; the numbers, types, and qualifications of the staff in the facility; and the financial status, resources, and considerations of the facilities and organizations involved. How adequate or inadequate these factors are will affect not only the quality of services and programs provided to the client, but also how well a facility or program complies with the standards of external regulatory laws and agencies and professional standards of practice.

## MEDICAL CHARTS AND RECORDS

While TRSs must conduct their own testing using TR/RT and other instruments they select as appropriate for each individual client as part of a comprehensive assessment process, they can also obtain necessary and valuable information from medical charts and related records. They have to utilize information that already exists, to eliminate having to "reinvent the wheel" by repeating recent assessments already made, and to obtain data reported by other disciplines, which they are not qualified to evaluate. For example, the TRS will find the medical diagnoses that physicians have determined from examining a client. These can include not only physiological illnesses, injuries, and conditions, but also diagnoses of mental health disorders and conditions made by psychiatrists and/or psychologists, and client personality analyses/psychological profiles by psychologists, which can inform TRS services selection. Healthcare records can include information reported by social service workers. PT and OT evaluation and service reports of previous/existing therapies and needs further inform TR/RT planning. In some healthcare facilities, activity therapists' reports about client activities and preferences also inform TRS assessment and planning.

## STAFF MEMBERS OF VARIOUS SETTINGS

In addition to administering assessment instruments used in the TR/RT field, TRSs also conduct assessments by obtaining data from other sources. Staff members in healthcare facilities, correctional facilities, school systems, etc., can be valuable sources of information about clients. For example, in nursing homes, they can get feedback from nurses about a client's daily behaviors, health status, and progress. They can find out from activity therapists whether a client has participated in any programmed activities and whether he or she has displayed any preferences/dislikes among activities. In school systems, TRSs can ask classroom teachers, special education teachers, educational specialists, other therapists, and paraprofessionals about students' recreational interests, adaptive devices, and classroom accommodations they need and use. They can ask PE teachers about how students participate in activities, games, sports, etc., including their strengths, weaknesses, preferences, and any required adaptations/accommodations/ modifications. In correctional facilities, counseling, psychological, activity, clerical, and guard staff as well as wardens can inform TRSs about inmate behavior, interests, goals, motivations, and activities. In psychiatric facilities, care staff as well as psychological staff can inform TRSs of client behaviors, cautions, triggers, motivators, reinforcers, and effective/ineffective approaches for interaction.

## CLIENT'S SUPPORT SYSTEM

When conducting a comprehensive client assessment, TRSs can frequently get much helpful information from **family members** about the client's developmental history, common behaviors, leisure and recreational preferences, and history of the client's medical conditions from a home perspective to supplement medical examinations, diagnoses, and reports. Parents, grandparents, siblings, spouses, children, and other family members usually know the client best and can offer personal insights not available to professional practitioners and other service providers. Some clients with disabilities also have advocates who help them obtain needed services and equipment; these **support persons** can inform TRSs of client needs as well as of resources to help meet those needs. Some clients and/or their caregivers are also members of various support groups. Representatives and members of these groups can help TRSs in a range of ways, including informing them of ongoing/frequent emotions the client has expressed; what types of respite and other support needs their caregivers have expressed, been observed to need, and received/not received; and specialized adaptive equipment and services the client has needed/used for specific disabilities or conditions.

## CONSIDERATIONS WHEN GATHERING DATA FROM A CLIENT'S SUPPORT SYSTEM

By gathering information from clients, their family members, caregivers, and other service providers, TRSs can learn of specific client characteristics and symptoms and associated precautions to take. For example, many individuals with seizure disorders experience auras (distinctive odors, sounds, lights, or other sensory phenomena) that signal an impending seizure. Some children and intellectually disabled adults may be identified as "runners" who unexpectedly bolt from the room or area. Clients with mental illnesses, substance abuse disorders, more commonplace neuroses, or simply adolescent age status may display resistant behaviors when confronting TRSs whom they perceive as authority figures and/or tasks they find challenging or intimidating. Family members and caregivers often have developed specific behavior management techniques, communication methods, and other "tricks" that are effective to encourage clients to take medications, perform daily living activities, comply with requests and rules, etc. Being informed of these can give TRSs valuable guidance. For clients with cerebral palsy, swimming in cold water and hearing sudden loud noises exacerbate spasticity. Clients with seizure disorders may become unable to follow spoken directions during seizure activity. Knowing these things can help TRSs take precautions against such impairments and symptoms.

## SELECTING ASSESSMENT METHODS

Different TR/RT assessments are designed for different purposes; TRSs will select different instruments according to their purposes for evaluation. For example, among leisure assessments, if a client is referred who has not participated in leisure activities before or after the current/recent diagnosis, the TRS would choose instruments to identify barriers to leisure activity and to define client attitudes toward leisure. Some examples include the Leisure Diagnostic Battery (LDB), Leisure Attitude Scale (LAS), Leisure Motivation Scale (LMS), Leisure Satisfaction Measure (LSM), and Life Satisfaction Scale (LSS). If a TRS wants to assess the previous leisure participation patterns of an adolescent client needing rehabilitation following an injury/illness, he or she could administer the Teen Leisurescope Plus and the State Technical Institute Leisure Assessment Process (STILAP). If a TRS wants to assess the functional abilities of a new client presenting with a diagnosis of a psychological disorder, he or she might use the Comprehensive Evaluation in Recreation Therapy–Psychiatric/Behavioral (CERT–PB). To assess what a new client with permanent physical disabilities can/cannot do for planning TR/RT activities, the CERT–PD for Physical Disabilities would apply.

## DETERMINING STRENGTHS AND LIMITATIONS OF ASSESSMENT INSTRUMENTS
### RELIABILITY

Reliability refers to whether a test can obtain consistent results from the same participants over repeated administrations. For example, if a TRS administers an assessment instrument suitable for group administration to a group of clients and then administers it again two weeks later, and the clients have not begun participating in any TR/RT treatments or activities in the interim, they should achieve the same or similar results on the instrument as they did the first time if the instrument is reliable, hence dependable. Some types of reliability include test-retest reliability, which the aforementioned example illustrates; equivalent-forms reliability; and internal consistency reliability. Equivalent-forms/alternate-forms reliability is demonstrated by giving two otherwise identical tests but with differing items and correlating both scores. This is used when alternate test forms are available and when participants are likely to remember their answers from the first administration. Internal consistency reliability involves determining how each the items on a test relate to all of its other items.

## VALIDITY

Validity refers to whether/how much a testing instrument measures what it intends and/or claims to measure, rather than something else.

- **Face validity** is how much a test intuitively seems on the face of it to measure what it says it does.
- **Content validity** is whether the entire area a test intends to measure is covered by the test's content. For example, a test of American geography should not contain only questions about the geography of the Midwestern states, but about all states in America.
- **Predictive validity** is how well a test's scores can predict its scores in a later administration.
- **Concurrent validity** is how well a test's scores relate to scores on an established other test/other valid measure given at the same time. For example, if one wants to replace an unwieldy test with a new, simpler one, administer both and compare results.
- **Construct validity** is how well a test measures some abstract/hypothetical concept or construct. Establishing construct validity helps to validate interpretations concerning a given construct.

## PRACTICALITY

Some assessment instruments may be very well-designed and have high degrees of statistically demonstrated validity and reliability, yet they may also be impractical. For example, an instrument that takes several hours to administer would not be practical to administer to clients with short attention spans, such as those with intellectual disabilities, attention deficit hyperactivity disorder, or traumatic brain injuries. Another practicality consideration can be that an assessment instrument requires 1:1 administration, but the setting where the assessment takes place does not have sufficient staffing to accommodate this requirement. Self-reporting instruments designed for clients with high cognitive functioning levels have no practical application for use with clients functioning at low cognitive levels. Instruments that are administered by having clients fill out written forms are impractical for clients who are illiterate or intellectually disabled. Computerized assessments have great advantages, but are impractical to administer with clients lacking computer literacy.

## AVAILABILITY

A TRS may know from exposure during education and/or previous employment that a particular assessment instrument is an excellent resource for evaluation; however, it may not be available in the TRS's current employment setting. Some excellent instruments are expensive to purchase from their publishers; some agencies or practices cannot afford these expenditures. In other instances, a certain setting may simply have different tests available for its employees to utilize routinely. The TRS might request that the employer procure an assessment instrument that he or she prefers and/or is more familiar with; employers that can afford to do so may agree, both to accommodate the employee request and, appreciating this new input, to expand their repertoire of available assessment instruments. However, other employers, even if they can afford additional tests, may refuse to honor such requests for various reasons. School systems typically use assessments approved by their districts and states to align with standards; this can affect test availability for TRSs employed in educational settings.

## SUMMARIZING THE CLIENT'S STRENGTHS AND NEEDS IN THE ASSESSMENT PROCESS

After a TRS has collected data, both objective and subjective, about a client from both primary and secondary sources in a comprehensive assessment, he or she will then develop a statement that summarizes current client functional status, strengths, and needs. Based on this statement, the TRS will write clinical impressions and recommendations for referral, intervention, or no service. The TRS will use this statement after assessment during planning, to guide sharing assessment results with client and family to identify goals they desire from intervention and determine goal priorities. The TRS often presents the statement of strengths, needs, and functional status to an interdisciplinary team of specialists from various fields during staffing events, such as meetings including the client, caregivers, and team members to develop interagency transitions and/or integrate services and programs. The TRS will also document the statement in the client's record. This statement is also used in planning inclusion programs to inform experience selections. The information in the TRS's statement constitutes baseline data for later assessing client progress and TR/RT plan effectiveness.

# Apply Assessment Data to Plan of Care

## APPLYING ASSESSMENT RESULTS TO THE PLANNING PROCESS

Assessment findings not only inform the TRS's planning and implementation of individual services and programs directly, as when certain assessment results provide diagnoses of an injury/illness/disability the treatment will address, they also inform the characteristics, methods, techniques, and strategies the TRS chooses for intervention, as when other assessment results provide diagnoses that will not be remediated by intervention but influence how it is delivered. For example, if a client is diagnosed with an intellectual, cognitive, behavioral, or other disability and the TRS has then assessed at what levels the client can pay attention, how long he or she can maintain attention, how long he or she takes to learn and remember new information, how long he or she can retain information, at what levels of complexity he or she can understand information, and how well he or she can follow directions, this will inform what kinds of activities the TRS plans; their complexity/simplicity levels, durations, repetitions; and what kinds of directions to give during intervention. Various psychological, intellectual, and other disabilities/characteristics also influence the therapeutic relationship and TRS-client interactions, guiding professional behavior according to the individual client.

## GOALS AND MEASURABLE OBJECTIVES

Goals should be achievable aims (essentially end results) developed for specific departments, the organization, groups of clients, or individual clients, focusing on improving performance. For example: "The client will engage in recreational activities with peers." Measurable objectives are the narrow steps taken to achieve wider goals. The elements that should be included in a measurable objective include:

- **Who**: Those who need to change in some way must be identified. These may include the nurses, physicians, clients, teams, or the organization as a whole.
- **Outcomes**: The desired outcomes must be clearly outlined.
- **Measure**: The method of assessing outcomes, including any tool, survey, data, demonstration, must be clear.
- **Level of proficiency**: Criteria determining success or failure should be clear.
- **Timeframe**: The time needed to achieve objectives should be stated.

Example: "At the end of 30 days, the client will participate in gym class ≥80% of the time."

## SMART Goals

### Specific

SMART stands for Specific, Measurable, Attainable, Realistic, and Timely. The **SMART system** is used in any discipline where people must create goals and objectives. This includes education; special education; psychology; behavior modification programs; health care; health and human services; treatment plans; therapy plans, including TR/RT plans; personal fitness plans; self-improvement services; business plans, etc. A goal or objective is much more likely to be attained if it is specific than if it is general. For example, making a goal (like some people make New Year's resolutions) to "get in shape" physically is an example of a goal that is too general. However, making a goal to "join a health club and work out three times a week" is more specific. "Walk faster" is too general; "walk one mile in 15 minutes" is more specific. To make a goal or objective specific, ask six "W" questions: *Who* is involved in this goal? *What* do I want to achieve? *Where* will I do this? *When* will I do this? *Which* constraints and requirements are involved in accomplishing this goal? *Why* do I want to achieve this goal (specific purposes, benefits, or reasons)?

### Measurable

Goals must not only be specific; they must also be measurable. In other words, one must be able to quantify a goal/objective, describing it with an action verb with a measurable result from the physical/cognitive/psychological/social/spiritual/leisure behavior domain, and the environment, activities, or other conditions pertinent to performing the action. Vague descriptions like "a lot" or "significantly" are not measurements. The criterion of measurability has its origin in behavioral psychology and behavior modification techniques. According to behaviorism, only outwardly observable behaviors that can be measured can be modified. Internal states/processes like thoughts, feelings, moods, decisions, etc., cannot be observed or measured and hence cannot be externally manipulated to change. To set measurable goals, determine criteria for attaining them, including number, frequency, duration, and success percentage as applicable (e.g., after 8 weeks in therapy, the client will ambulate using a wheelchair for at least 10 minutes with only two rest breaks, twice per day, 90% of the time).

### Attainable

Goals must not only be specific in nature, not general, and measurable; they must also be attainable. This means that the person for whom the goal is written—oneself, or one's client, patient, or student—actually has the ability to achieve the goal. For example, a person who sustained a massive brain injury may never be able to perform intellectually in the same way that he or she could before the injury; but he or she may eventually be able to regain many functional abilities for independent or supported daily living. An individual who had both legs amputated may never be able to set or break a world record for running a race with the fastest time, but may be able to walk and even run races using state-of-the-art prostheses with enough rehabilitation and training.

### Realistic

Goals must not only be defined specifically, possible to measure numerically, and attainable by the person who will be pursuing the goal, but also realistic. For example, a TRS writes a goal for a client receiving TR/RT as part of rehabilitation for a minor injury to acquire several new leisure skills; this would be realistic, but the same goal for a client receiving TR/RT within rehabilitation for a massive major injury would be unrealistic: the client must first regain enough basic functional skills for daily living activities before acquiring new leisure skills. SMART criteria are interrelated (e.g., "A" attainable/achievable and "T" timely/time-bound must be jointly realistic). In the aforementioned example, some goals for the client with the minor injury would not be attainable for the client with the major injury (e.g., if that injury caused paralysis). A six-week time frame, appropriate for the client with the minor injury, would be inappropriate for the client with the major injury, who might need a year or longer.

## TIMELY

Goals must also be timely/time-bound; to write a clearly defined goal, one must include how long it should take to achieve it. In addition to a total duration, one should specify the beginning and ending dates of the goal. The time frame established must be realistic for the goal specified. A TRS would use knowledge of the usual/average/typical times to achieve certain activities plus knowledge of the individual client's current status, limitations, motivations, and abilities to estimate time and adjust this criterion as needed according to the client's progress.

# Planning

## Develop Individualized Plan of Care

### ELEMENTS OF AN INDIVIDUALIZED INTERVENTION PLAN

The individualized treatment plan for the therapeutic recreation client may vary and may be a combined assessment and treatment plan in some cases. However, elements usually found in the treatment plan include:

- Description of the client's disability or rehabilitation problem.
- Client's goal.
- Short and long-term goals of therapy (increased cognitive, physical, socialization/emotional skills, leisure education, participation in recreational activities).
- Short and long-term objectives: Cognitive (improve concentration, memory activities, problem solving, communication skills, academic skills), physical (increase strength, endurance, fine or gross motor skills, practice relaxation, fall prevention, balance exercises), and socialization/emotional (adjustment to disabilities, social skills, improve self-image, increases ability to communicate and express feelings).
- Purpose of leisure education.
- Purpose of participation in recreational activities.
- Precautions or any contraindications for activities or services.
- List of current medications and possible adverse effects.
- Need for assistive technology or adapted equipment.
- Methods/Interventions to be utilized (structured activities, exploration, independent activities, community reintegration).

### AWARENESS OF CLIENT CONTRAINDICATIONS

Through positive communication practices, TRSs can develop awareness of certain therapeutic experiences that are contraindicated for a particular client and enter these into the client's individual program plan (IPP). For example, some medications that lower high blood pressure can cause dizziness, so TRSs avoid activities with greater risks for falling and note this side effect in the records to inform other practitioners. Some drugs can cause dizziness upon standing up from sitting; TRSs avoid orthostatic testing and therapeutic activities involving standing up quickly and are prepared to catch swaying/listing/toppling clients. Certain medical conditions and antipsychotic drugs can cause tremors, precluding activities requiring precise fine-motor control. Clients taking anticonvulsants for seizure disorders may not notice or display medication side effects in medical settings, but when they expend greater energy during community outings, symptoms become more noticeable to them and others. Anti-seizure medications often cause sleepiness, so TRSs and other providers must be aware of client alertness levels during activities to avoid accidents/injuries. Various medications can impair coordination, contraindicating activities demanding complex, skilled movements, speed, agility, etc.

## SERVICE DELIVERY MODELS

### MAIN CATEGORIES OF HEALTHCARE SERVICE DELIVERY SYSTEMS

Healthcare services can be classified by complexity and types of services into the following:

- **Health promotion and illness prevention**: Since the 1980s, the historically dominant perspective of disease treatment has gradually shifted to one of health promotion. Health promotion service programs include smoking cessation, stress management, weight control, physical activity, healthy diets, etc. Such programs and activities are found in various settings. Illness prevention services, involving communities or individual patients, include offering vaccinations; identifying risk factors for diabetes, cardiovascular disease, and other illnesses; assisting people in preventing such illnesses; and environmental programs, often government-mandated, to prevent illnesses.
- **Diagnosis and treatment**: Diagnosing and treating illness has occupied the greatest part of healthcare systems. In addition to physician practices and hospitals, community clinics have recently also become service providers of early cancer detection education and mammograms. Some shopping center/mall walk-in clinics offer cholesterol, blood sugar, and other diagnostic screenings.
- **Rehabilitation**: Rehabilitation is the process of restoring people to previous/possible health levels and useful physical, psychological, social, and vocational functions.

### MEDICAL MODEL

The medical model is the oldest treatment model. Service delivery is modeled after principles and methods of the medical profession. Conditions are regarded and treated as medical illnesses/diseases. Evaluation typically includes laboratory analysis of physiological testing; treatment often includes medication. A summary of the historical basis of this model emphasizes main elements of symptom, diagnosis, treatment, and cure. Physicians and other service providers have the role of treating disease conditions. The medical model has been applied to the mental health, social casework, alcoholism and addictions, and corrections fields. With respect to TR/RT, the medical health and human services model dictates that the physician is the primary practitioner who determines the roles of TRSs and others involved in treatment. This model assumes the client is a patient with an illness to be healed, cured, or treated. The medical model disregards the client's holistic needs and focuses on the disease condition. The doctor's diagnosis/diagnoses and prescription(s) guide the course of TR/RT. The medical model is typically applied in medical hospitals, surgical hospitals, clinics, physical medicine and rehabilitation settings.

### COMMUNITY MODEL

The community model of health and human services delivery, with respect to TR/RT, may also be known as the *special recreation model*. According to this model, TR/RT service includes a critical element of providing a wide variety of leisure opportunities within the client's community. Therefore, the TRS should provide clients with opportunities to choose among the experiences they have and the skills they learn to enable them to participate in community-based programs of leisure and recreational activities. In the second half of the 20th century, TR and other health and human services were affected by deinstitutionalization when services to persons with disabilities were shifted from public facilities to the communities, increasing the need for community-based services. Some of the settings where activities based on the special recreation or community model of health and human services delivery can be found include programs offered by the National Easter Seal Society; the American Foundation for the Blind; the United Cerebral Palsy Association; the ARC; and city, county, or other municipal recreation departments.

## EDUCATIONAL OR TRAINING MODEL

The educational or training model of delivering health and human services emphasizes helping clients to acquire the knowledge and skills they will need to become productive members of society who can make contributions. Accordingly, with such an orientation, this model of service delivery has a strong focus on a structure similar to the educational classroom. With respect to TR/RT services, this model includes teaching both leisure skills and social skills to its participants. The education and training model of health and human services delivery also places strong emphasis upon providing vocational training, remedial education, and occupational therapy (OT). Because individuals with developmental disabilities frequently need multiple training in social skills, vocational and workplace skills, remedial levels of education, and OT to improve and refine their fine motor skills for performing both activities of daily living and occupational tasks, the education or training model of service delivery is often applied with this population. This model is typically followed in practices found in sheltered workshops for persons with intellectual and other developmental disabilities, vocational rehabilitation and habilitation centers, schools, and daycare centers.

## PSYCHOSOCIAL REHABILITATION MODEL

Compared to other, older models like the medical model, community model, and education or training model of health and human service delivery, the psychosocial rehabilitation model is a more recent development. This model distinguishes mental illnesses from other, physiological illnesses in the sense that although some physiological conditions are chronic, others are curable and hence temporary, whereas mental illness is most often chronic—either continuous or recurrent—and that therefore, it is inappropriate to apply the medical model to the treatment of patients suffering from persistent, severe mental disorders. The orientation of this model is to examine the abilities and strengths of the client and make use of these and to remain in the here and now rather than dwell on the past. The goal of the psychosocial rehabilitation model is to promote the client's optimal level of functioning in the community, which includes participating in activities as well as residing there. To realize this goal, practitioners help their clients to acquire education, vocational skills, social skills, coping skills, personal adaptation skills, recreational skills, and household living and maintenance skills.

## HEALTH AND WELLNESS MODEL

The historical orientation of health and human service delivery was from the perspective of disease, typified by the medical model of diagnosing and treating illnesses. However, in recent years this perspective has shifted to health and wellness. The emphasis has changed toward preventing illness before it occurs through practices promoting wellness; nutritious diets; avoiding harmful habits like smoking tobacco, overindulging in alcohol, and eating junk foods high in sodium, saturated fats, and refined sugar and flour; regular wellness doctor visits; regular wellness and prevention tests; mammograms, PAP smears, prostate examinations, hernia checks, vision and hearing tests, cancer screenings, etc. Along with emphasizing wellness over illness, realization has increased of the relationship between individual and community health. The World Health Organization's ICF and US Department of Health and Human Services' Healthy People initiatives reflect this holistic approach. TR/RT has adopted this perspective by applying cross-cultural and interdisciplinary communication to further positive growth and integrating economic responsibility with evidence-based results, making interventions both briefer and more effective, continually improving and documenting service safety and quality.

## PERSON-CENTERED MODEL

The person-centered model of health and human services delivery regards the client not as an illness or a disorder, but rather as a whole person with specific preferences, gifts, and strengths.

88

This model finds a key requirement to health is the practitioner's recognizing, understanding, and working with the individual's cultural, language, and ethnic preferences in their service provision. Person-centered services help decrease client dependence on the system while promoting client community living, engagement of natural client supports, and meaningful client involvement in recovery and a fulfilling life. Clients are viewed not as passive patients or service recipients, but active experts in their own lives who take responsibility for directing their own wellness processes and engage provider expertise to assist them. Rather than providing services as separate instances responding to crises, person-centered care management models emphasize continuing, constructive, flexible relationships, which anticipate needs when possible and meet them as they develop. The person-centered model is a comprehensive approach to understanding every individual and his or her family's history, shared strengths, needs, culture, spirituality, and healing. Service plans and results are based on respect for the whole person's unique dignity, strengths, and preferences.

## RECOVERY MODEL

When applying the recovery model to a client with mental illness, the planning goal is to allow clients to maintain control of their lives (even when they can't control their symptoms) and to make decisions rather than focusing on returning to previous levels of functioning (which may or may not be realistic). Self-determination is central to this model, and clients should begin planning when desired even though the clients may not be fully recovered (or may never fully recover). The recovery model focuses on the skills and resilience the clients have and encourages them to establish new goals and move forward with life, recognizing that clients' recovery is influenced by the attitudes and expectations of others and the support system available to the clients. This model recognizes that a supportive environment includes adequate financial resources, relationships with others, and rewarding work. Clients need to feel they are listened to, respected, and understood. Clients should be aware of community resources and provided the tools to access these resources.

## HUMAN SERVICES DELIVERY SYSTEMS

Health, education, and social services are commonly included within human services. It is also common to combine health services and other human services into one category, as in the US Department of Health and Human Services (HHS). Decentralization is a major aspect of the American educational system. Whereas US states carry most of the legal authority in educational services, operational matters are decided largely by the thousands of local school districts nationwide. State and local governments provide far more public school funding than the federal government. Public concerns over education include achievement gaps in a society that is rapidly becoming more demographically diverse. Parents, educators, legislators, and others have also been concerned that increased government expenditures invested in educational funding have not commensurately increased student achievement. While overall dropout rates have decreased, not only are they still considered excessive, they also have more serious consequences today than in earlier times, when more unskilled jobs were available. Today, more occupations require greater literacy. Economic problems, inadequate teacher pay, and school program and instructional quality contribute to inadequate student performance. School reform initiatives call for systemic changes, including integrating educational and non-educational needs.

### SERVICES INCORPORATED INTO HUMAN SERVICES

Human services typically incorporate health, education, and social services. However, our federal government separates education but combines health and social services by department. Like education, the social services delivery system is decentralized, but more so. Federal, state, and local governments fund social services, and consumers additionally buy social services from many providers with comparatively narrow scope. Consistent information regarding services and recipients is not available nationwide due to the variety of for-profit, nonprofit, local, and state government agencies providing them. The social services system tries to meet a wide array of needs. Despite these efforts, many children and families live in poverty in a nation containing great wealth. The social services system is unable to protect many children from abuse, neglect, and/or homelessness and provide them with care. The size of the United States, the fragmented nature of the system, multiple organizations, varying attributes of social services professionals, insufficient resources, and changing societal composition and hence demands, contribute to these inadequacies despite organizations' motivation for innovation and collaboration, which is also impeded by insufficient leadership capacities.

## LEISURE ABILITY MODEL

The Leisure Ability model of TR/RT may be the most frequently used model today for delivering TR/RT services. It is also among the oldest TR/RT models. Its assumption is that gratifying leisure functioning, enhancing a person's independence, directly improves happiness and quality of life as the main result of TR/RT services. Theoretical influences on the conceptual foundations of the Leisure Ability model include internal locus of control, internalized motivation, freedom of choice, personal causality, and optimal experiences or flow. TRSs utilize functional intervention, recreational participation, and leisure education to enable satisfying, independent client leisure functioning and lifestyles. Interventions target physical, mental, emotional, and social functional skills required for leisure and other life participation and experiences. TRSs accomplish pre-identified client changes/improvements by carefully designing and selecting facilitative techniques and skills. Leisure education develops knowledge, skills, and attitudes expanding client participation capacities. Recreation participation services involve organized, structured programs enabling client practice and application of skills and knowledge acquired during functional intervention and leisure education. Clients take responsibility for decision-making, behavioral self-regulation, and participation results, while TRSs serve as instructors, leaders, supervisors, facilitators, advisors, and/or counselors.

## LEISURE SERVICES SYSTEM

The leisure services system is responsible to sponsor parks, recreation, and other leisure facilities and programs available to the public. Ten types of provider organizations in today's society delivering leisure services are: (1) public agencies; (2) nonprofit organizations; (3) commercial recreation enterprises; (4) employee service and recreation programs offered by employing companies; (5) the US Armed Forces; (6) private membership organizations; (7) campus recreational programs offered at colleges and universities; (8) therapeutic recreation/recreational therapy services; (9) sports management organizations; and (10) leisure and recreational programs offered by the hospitality and tourism industry. **Characteristics of public and government agencies** that provide leisure services include the following:

- The main source of support for most government and public leisure and recreation agencies has been money obtained through taxes.
- Governmental leisure service agencies consider themselves as being primarily responsible for serving the recreational needs of the public and forming the core of the recreation movement.
- Government agency responsibility for managing our natural resources goes hand-in-hand with recreational management, exemplified in thousands of Parks and Recreation Departments nationwide.

## HEALTH PROTECTION/HEALTH PROMOTION MODEL

According to the Health Protection/Health Promotion model, TR/RT has the purpose of both protecting health (helping people recover after their health has been threatened) and promoting health (helping people to attain the highest level of health that they can). Basic assumptions of this model are that all humans have intrinsic drives to pursue and maintain wellness and health; that therapeutic relationships with TRSs can help to realize these instincts; and that TRSs accomplish this realization through structuring prescriptive recreational activities, mutual participation in recreation by clients and therapists, and self-directed client leisure activity, which the therapist has facilitated by instructing the client in leisure skills, access, and preference identification and guiding/supporting self-direction. According to David Austin, author of a leading health protection/health promotion model, TR/RT services should focus on encouraging clients not merely to recover from illness but to attain optimal health. Theoretical concepts underlying this model include humanistic psychology, incorporating human tendencies to actualization and stabilization; high wellness levels; and health. Both adaptive coping and personal growth and development comprise health. TR/RT's application of suitable leisure and recreation experiences helps protect and promote health.

### COMPONENTS

Austin (1998) distinguishes between health protection and health promotion thusly: Health protection involves rehabilitation or treatment of disability or illness, whereas health promotion is oriented to wellness. Health protection is motivated to restore former health; health promotion is motivated to improve health status. In this model, TR/RT is perceived as both concerned with relieving and preventing illness similarly to traditional, medically-oriented allied health professions, and also collaboratively practicing "well medicine" with physicians to help clients to attain optimal wellness, health, and self-actualization. Clients identify themselves by desiring better health. TRSs serve to further client attainment of independence and control. The model's mission is to enable recovery, or adaptive coping, and optimal health. Austin has advocated expanding his model to include the use of TR/RT to help clients cope with chronic disabilities/illnesses, prevent/decrease further deterioration, and/or improve quality of life to reach the highest realistic health levels possible for them rather than cure them when this is unrealistic. The model moves through a continuum of three main components: prescriptive activities, recreation, and leisure. TRS direction progressively decreases/client direction increases as health improves.

## TR SERVICE DELIVERY MODEL

In the TR Service Delivery model, the scope of TR/RT services includes (1) a needs assessment or diagnosis; (2) rehabilitation or treatment for a need or problem; (3) educational services; and (4) activities for prevention and health promotion. Initially, the client provides informed consent to receive services. Through the course of treatment, the client moves toward greater autonomy until he or she becomes self-sufficient and can make informed choices. TRS interventions enable client change; clients become empowered to attain their goals. (1) involves formal evaluation, using assessment instruments appropriate to individual client abilities, strengths, and limitations. (2) involves interventions with purposes, direct and/or indirect, of remediating injury/disease effects, primary and/or secondary and restoring abilities/functions. As examples, exercise produces endorphins which alleviate mild client depression; cognitive retraining can improve attention span and memory in clients with brain injuries. Self-care, stress management, and other skills and techniques are taught through education. Prevention and health promotion foster and reinforce healthy lifestyle behaviors to improve/maintain functioning and/or wellbeing. This model's intervention dimension involves TRS actions and client efforts to attain specific therapeutic goals. Its experiential dimension emphasizes leisure states of mind, proceeding from perceived freedom and internal motivation and producing satisfaction and joy.

## TRS-CLIENT INTERACTION

Although the TRS-client interaction is complex and individualized, some generalized principles can inform understanding of TR/RT service delivery. According to Van Andel's TR Service Delivery model, the nature of the TRS-client interaction will to some extent be determined by the predominating service philosophy. For example, in acute-care centers subscribing to the medical model, the patient will be subordinate to the therapist, whereas in community settings, the client's need for independence and autonomy will be reinforced. The nature of the individual client impairment will also influence the therapist-client relationship. While humane care principles require giving all clients as much autonomy as possible to decide how they will participate and which services they need, clients with more severe impairments are often more dependent on others for decision-making regarding their healthcare needs. TRS-client interactions pursue the ultimate goal of client independence. The therapist-client interaction will also be influenced by the type of service. Therapists generally use more directive approaches when conducting needs assessments and treatments, which are more based on the medical model, than when providing preventive or educational services. Still, informing clients adequately about expected results and the nature of services can (and should) prevent therapist-client authority-dependency relationships.

## HOLISTIC MODEL

Traditional approaches to health based on the medical model focused on specific illnesses or injuries and treating them. In recent decades, newer approaches have begun to replace this perspective, viewing health not as resolution or absence of pathology but a complete state of physical, mental, and social wellness. Rather than concentrating only on the condition/symptoms, practitioners now more often consider the whole person—hence the term holistic (or wholistic). This attitude is being reflected throughout many health and human services fields. For example, leisure is not a separately compartmentalized component of life, but an experience found in all aspects of life. On a broader level, TR/RT is now viewed as a holistic process, not restricted to certain treatment/activity settings or groups of people; it can apply to anybody in any setting whose goals and needs could benefit from TR/RT interventions. As a holistic process, TR/RT deliberately applies recreational and experiential interventions to effect physical, intellectual, emotional, social, and/or spiritual changes that can improve and/or maintain health, functional performance, and quality of life.

## INTERDISCIPLINARY APPROACH TO THE HOLISTIC PERSPECTIVE

A holistic perspective regarding health and human services requires serving the whole person rather than separately treating isolated disease conditions, for example, because these are all interrelated. Similarly, human services like economic assistance, concrete services, nutrition assistance, nutritional counseling, etc., are interrelated. Individuals and families in need more often require several or all of these services rather than just one. In an interdisciplinary approach, a TRS collaborates with other professions in treating the client as a whole person. For example, a client who is recovering from an accident causing bone fractures and muscle sprains may have surgery performed by an orthopedist. Once this physician finds the fractures have healed, he or she may refer the patient for physical therapy to rehabilitate the soft tissue damage, restore mobility and range of motion, and restore or approximate the person's previous levels of physical functioning. The physical therapist may find that the patient has a limited repertoire of leisure activities and refer him or her for TR/RT as an adjunct and complement to physical therapy.

## STRENGTHS-BASED APPROACH, PERSON-CENTERED APPROACH, AND PALLIATIVE CARE

Approaches utilized by the recreation therapist include:

- **Strength-based approach**: Focuses on strengths and abilities of the client rather than deficits and disabilities. Program decisions are based on the capabilities of the client. The focus of this approach is on the whole person rather than isolated problems.
- **Person-centered**: The client's autonomy is central to decision-making and the RT works collaboratively with the client to ensure that the goals of the client are the basis for the treatment plan. The RT should plan leisure activities that correspond to the client's preferences.
- **Palliative care**: The focus of therapy is to improve the quality of the client's life and to relieve pain and discomfort. Palliative care services may include educating the client about available programs and providing information about transportation services and other community resources. Clients may benefit from exercise programs to increase strength, improve balance, and prevent falls.

## TR/RT MODELS FOR VARIOUS SETTINGS

### HOSPITALS

In some hospitals, most of the TR/RT programs offered involve general recreation. The reasons for this can be ratios of patients to staff much larger than is ideal, which occurs frequently; professional staff who have lower levels of preparation; or in some cases, the institutional philosophy. For example, some nursing facilities regard their primary function as care, whether acute or long-term, rather than as rehabilitation of patients. Another consideration related to TR/RT practice in hospitals is its function for limiting the length of hospital stays for patients. Historically, hospitals or institutions were the sites of all TR/RT services provided. However, over time, trends toward enabling community living for persons with disabilities by providing community-based services and programs, combined with increased requirements for facility accountability, the global nature of care, and the prohibitively high cost of hospital care have resulted in one application of hospital TR/RT for the purpose of returning patients to homes and communities. Still, medical facilities continue to be settings where many CTRSs practice.

### LONG-TERM CARE FACILITIES

Elderly people with impairments related to aging are often placed in residential assisted living facilities. Other long-term care facilities include skilled nursing facilities, where people of all ages with serious chronic conditions are served. While the recent trend in mental health facilities has been markedly toward brief service and discharge, some patients with chronic mental disorders may still receive care of a more long-term nature there. In any of these settings, TRSs are often employed to provide services related to both rehabilitation and ongoing needs for therapeutic recreation interventions; regular opportunities to engage in structured recreational activities; and instruction in leisure education areas including learning, developing, and applying leisure skills; expanding repertoires of leisure skills and activities; learning about where and how to access leisure resources and opportunities in the future as a part of transition and discharge planning; and learning how to identify their individual strengths and preferences and select suitable leisure activities accordingly.

### COMMUNITY RECREATION SETTINGS

While many TRSs are employed in healthcare facilities like hospitals, rehabilitation centers, mental health facilities, skilled nursing facilities, assisted living and other long-term care facilities, and residential transitional facilities for persons with developmental disabilities, many others practice in community-based settings. These include school systems, day habilitation centers and outpatient day treatment centers, halfway houses for individuals recovering from substance abuse or mental health disorders, and community-based recreation programs administered by parks and recreation departments, adult day habilitation centers specialized for certain needs, adaptive sport centers for consumers with various disabilities, and different nonprofit agencies. In some senses, TRSs provide TR/RT services in any setting where a need for services exists and is identified. Community-based, inclusive human service programs such as horseback riding, camping, river running, water skiing, other outdoor adventure experiences, and adaptive sports programs all employ TR/RT professionals. Changing societal needs, healthcare reform, and healthcare technological advances require TRSs to network with community agencies. Community-based settings need little equipment or technical support. The 1963 Community Mental Health Centers and 1965 Older Americans Acts mandate more community-based than residential services, including TR/RT.

## HOME HEALTH CARE

Aspects of TR/RT service in the home health care environment include assessing the client's ability to restore function and to rehabilitate, assessing the home environment for safety and support systems, assessing the community for resources to aid the client's development, and assisting the client to carry out activities to improve health and wellbeing. Services may include:

- Improving the client's ability to communicate with others.
- Helping the client to attain confidence and improved ability in interpersonal skills.
- Improving the client's cognitive skills.
- Encouraging and assisting the client to engage in appropriate recreational activities.
- Establishing a program to strengthen and improve motor skills.
- Reducing the risk of falls through strengthening and environmental safety measures.
- Improving the client's body awareness.
- Encouraging the client to express personal thoughts and feelings.
- Advocating for the client's right to autonomy and self-direction.
- Assisting the client to access community resources, including public transportation.

## CORRECTIONAL FACILITIES

More than half of US male prison inmates are incarcerated for violent offenses. Female inmates more often serve time for nonviolent offenses. Even though the majority of correctional supervision is over paroled offenders and those on community-based probation, still more Americans are incarcerated than released yearly, with numbers continuing to increase in recent decades. Functioning characteristics of prisoners include low self-esteem; poor judgment; difficulty managing interpersonal interactions and daily living activities; family conflict; antisocial behaviors; impaired impulse control; sensation-seeking; substance abuse; poor physical health; learned helplessness; social stigma and devaluation; anxiety, depression, and suicide; sports underachievement; and deficient leisure skills. TRSs provide inmates with experiences promoting self-awareness and higher self-esteem; better wellness, social skills, family leadership, and decision-making; resource awareness; stress management; coping with gang pressures and authority; management of discretionary time; and building vocational and academic skills. TR/RT relieves confinement's stresses, facilitates necessary exercise, and enables some freedom of choice. TR/RT services develop inmates' functional skills, cognitive skills, emotional control, anger management, and coping skills.

## CONSIDERATIONS FOR PROGRAMS IN CORRECTIONAL FACILITIES

Program content and settings are affected by safety and security concerns. Within the prison's limited personal freedom, systems of graduated privileges promote self-determination, enable some choice, and support acceptable amounts of self-expression and nonconformity. Weight lifting and other physical activities release tension; aerobics, jogging, volleyball, and basket-ball also release aggression via striking acceptable targets and rapid movements. Some prisons partner with animal shelters in programs wherein inmates care for and rehabilitate dogs for adoption, affording animal-assisted therapy and responsibility in caring for others. Recreation experiences involving inmates and family like holiday/ cultural events foster resiliency skills like tolerance and resource awareness. Families are empowered as active intervention team members. Adventure/challenge programs further inmate self-know-ledge, understanding of interpersonal interactions, self-determination, social capital, and positive youth development through immediate, concrete feedback and successful challenge completion. On-going youth challenges are addressed by individualized, holistic approaches, service continuity, and long-term intervention in supportive environments with role models. TRSs recognize inmate anger-management and social-skill deficits and perceptions of TRSs as authority figures, and avoid inmate devaluation. Voluntary inmate responsibilities improve self-esteem.

## WHO INTERNATIONAL CLASSIFICATION OF FUNCTIONING, DISABILITY, AND HEALTH

The World Health Organization (WHO) produced the International Classification of Functioning, Disability and Health (ICF). WHO's Family of International Classifications, mandated by its constitution, enables global consensus for a useful, meaningful structure and language that governments, providers, and consumers worldwide can commonly apply. Internationally accepted classifications for a variety of world settings enable comparing population data simultaneously and longitudinally; compiling nationally and internationally consistent data; and easier data storage, retrieval, analysis, and interpretation. This family includes the International Classification of Diseases (ICD), International Classification of Health Interventions (ICHI), and ICF. ICF is WHO's framework to measure health and disability on individual and population levels. All WHO member states endorsed ICF officially as the international standard for describing and measuring health and disability at the 2001 World Health Assembly. Because individual functioning and disability transpire in context, ICF also lists environmental factors. The WHO Disability Assessment Schedule is a practical instrument to measure general ICF-based health and disability levels. The ICF Checklist is a tool for time-efficiently, simply obtaining and recording information on individual functioning and disability. ICF Core Sets offer lists of health condition-specific and healthcare context-specific categories, enabling practical ICF application and user-friendly functioning and disability description.

## NORMALIZATION

Historically, persons with all types of disabilities—physical disabilities, intellectual disabilities, psychiatric disorders, etc.—were placed in institutions or hospital facilities. While a significant part of this policy was related to having medical personnel, equipment, medication, treatment and therapy programs, and direct care staff necessary to care adequately for the needs of individuals with serious disabilities, another contributing factor was the prevailing societal attitude of segregating people with disabilities from mainstream society. Some believed limitations prevented them from being productive, contributing members of society; others simply did not want to see persons with obvious differences/problems in appearance, function, and behavior in the community and everyday life. Some individuals with intellectual/mental/emotional/behavioral disabilities already had unusual behaviors—some simply attracting unwanted attention, others requiring extraordinary management efforts; some developed new/additional "institutionalized" behaviors from living in restricted environments surrounded by other abnormal behaviors. With legally mandated deinstitutionalization, normalization became a central concept for integrating people with disabilities into communities. They could not merely be placed in residences; they must be taught social, household management, job, and other skills. The goal became to enable persons with disabilities to live "normal"/"as normal as possible" lives.

## INCLUSION

Children with disabilities were traditionally educated in separate schools or classes pursuant to the idea that special education could best meet special needs. While this may have been based on good intentions to provide them the best educations, people with disabilities were denied access to public facilities, activities, and programs based on the assumption they would be unable to participate. This was originally true because facilities and activities were not designed to accommodate their physical, mental, or behavioral needs. When societal attitudes changed and laws were enacted to prevent discrimination against persons with disabilities, inclusion in mainstream education and society became a new directive. Children with disabilities have increasingly been educated in mainstream schools and classrooms. Laws require public facilities to eliminate architectural and other barriers. A significant way the inclusion trend has affected people with disabilities and TRSs is the federal mandate to enable all citizens' participation in community recreation programs. Public parks and recreation departments required to offer comprehensive services employ TRSs to design and implement inclusive recreation programs. Legally required transition plans included in student IEPs can include post-school community recreational activities. Professional organizations/conferences have provided TRS courses/training supporting incorporating recreation as a related service.

### CHARACTERISTICS OF INCLUSIVE RECREATION

One way in which the Americans with Disabilities Act (ADA) intended to stop discrimination against persons with disabilities was to support their inclusion in all parts of life, including recreation. Inclusive experiences acknowledge people's diversity and enable them to make choices based on abilities and preferences. TRSs plan TR/RT programs that include both people with and without disabilities. They may write individual inclusion plans for certain clients. They identify, procure, and assist clients in procuring adaptive equipment they will need to participate in certain recreational activities. They make task analyses of skill instruction to enable some clients to learn identified recreational skills. Administrators may provide inclusion assistants and companions to TRSs to help implement their programs. Inclusive programs and services must consider whether every type of client can be included, whether all personnel are prepared for including everybody, and must collaborate with other disciplines to facilitate the participation of clients with a variety of needs.

### NATIONAL RECREATION AND PARK ASSOCIATION POSITION STATEMENT ON INCLUSION

According to the National Recreation and Park Association Position Statement (1999) on Inclusion, all human beings have a right to pursue leisure, which it identifies as "a condition necessary for human dignity and wellbeing." This document also identifies that healthy leisure lifestyles promote wellness, prevent illness, enable personal self-direction and sense of competence, afford social interactions, and allow individual choice, contributing to the quality of life. Moreover, it states that people are entitled to take advantage of services and opportunities in the "most inclusive setting." They have the right to choose among the entire number of recreation opportunities that are available in various environments and settings and which require various levels of ability. This position statement includes a section on barrier removal. It stipulates that environments should be designed so as to promote acceptance, choice, risk-taking, fun, personal accomplishment, social interaction and cooperation, and that "physical barriers should be eliminated to facilitate full participation by individuals with disabilities."

### NATIONAL AND INTERNATIONAL INITIATIVES PROMOTING INCLUSION

In addition to laws like the ADA, which supports inclusion while prohibiting discrimination against persons with disabilities, the US Department of Health and Human Services (HHS) **Healthy People** initiatives, begun in 1979 for 1980–1990 and updated in Healthy People 2000, 2010, 2020 and

2030 not only promote proactive practices for good health and disease prevention, but also support providing inclusive services in American communities to enable access to health care, physical activity, good nutrition, etc. The **World Health Organization** (WHO) also promotes health and disease prevention for all people, incorporating inclusive community services, through its many initiatives, programs, research, and publications. TRSs and managers of businesses and other organizations provide recreation staff, people with and without disabilities, aides, and volunteers with in-service training to facilitate inclusion. They also develop individual inclusion plans, furnish adaptive equipment, use task analysis to instruct people in recreational and other skills, and provide inclusion assistants and companions to recreational programmers. The inclusion process follows steps reminiscent of APIE in TR/RT. Assessment questions include whether everybody can be included, feels welcome, and is prepared for inclusion.

## ACCESSIBILITY AND UNIVERSAL DESIGN

Accessibility involves designing and constructing facilities and areas, including public ones, in such a way that people with disabilities are able to use them and their resources. Accessibility applies not only to the physical properties of a place or facility, but more widely to programs and attitudes. A related term, universal design, means that architects and builders create environments including options for *all* people, disabled and nondisabled, to gain access in all manners. For example, a pathway with universal design would be accessible not only to people walking but also those using wheelchairs, riding bicycles, riding motor scooters, or pushing/sitting in baby carriages/strollers. Accessibility affects most people at least temporarily, and some permanently. The 1968 Architectural Barriers Act (PL 90–480) first required public buildings and facilities to be free of obstacles for people with disabilities. Section 504 of PL 93–112, the 1973 Vocational Rehabilitation Act Amendments, not only formed the Architectural and Transportation Barriers Compliance Board to enforce ABA compliance, but additionally extended accessibility to include program access. The 1990 Americans with Disabilities Act (ADA) strengthened the earlier laws.

## THEORIES OF PRACTICE
### BEHAVIORAL THEORY

Psychoanalytic theories, based on Freud's original psychodynamic theory or on neo-Freudian variations, rely on "talk therapy" wherein the patient explores the unconscious reasons for his or her feelings and behaviors. Because Freud believed our motivations were largely unconscious and the keys to our behaviors, this type of therapy is in-depth and time-consuming. Psychoanalysts listen, take notes, ask probing and guiding questions, and provide analyses of patient thoughts, emotions, and dreams. While patients can gain profound insights, they do not usually realize rapid change. In contrast, behavior modification measures outwardly observable behaviors and manipulates environmental events to change these by rewarding desired behaviors and punishing undesired ones. Participants experience more rapid changes in what they do regardless of understanding/not understanding why. Humanistic theorists and therapists disagree with the determinism of psychoanalysis and behaviorism, seeing human potential more optimistically. Carl Rogers' person-centered therapy provides clients with unconditional acceptance, reflective listening, and empathy to help them realize their full potential and works to align the ideal selves they wish to be with the real selves they are to enable self-actualization.

> **Review Video: Psychoanalytic Approach**
> Visit mometrix.com/academy and enter code: 162594

### PRINCIPLES AND APPLICATIONS

Behaviorism maintains that to change any behavior, it must first be outwardly observable and measurable. It is impossible to say a behavior has changed without measuring its original/baseline parameters (*frequency*, *intensity*, *duration*) and comparing those to measurements following intervention. Behavior modification manipulates *antecedents* and *consequences* to change specified behaviors. Antecedents likely to prompt desired behaviors are presented; antecedents likely to trigger undesired behaviors are prevented. Consequences increasing the probability of repeating a behavior are *reinforcements*; consequences decreasing it are *punishments*. *Positive reinforcement* presents a desired stimulus; *negative reinforcement* removes an undesired stimulus. Desired behaviors are made more frequent by repeatedly rewarding them until they become habits. *Extinction* eventually eliminates a behavior by removing reinforcement. The *Premack Principle* entails pairing an undesirable behavior with a desirable one, reinforcing and making the undesirable activity more desirable. *Shaping* reinforces *successive approximations* toward the behavior ultimately desired. *Chaining* reinforces one step at a time, adding successive steps in sequence to teach complex tasks in increments. This can be done as *forward chaining* starting with the first step or *backward chaining* starting with the last step.

## ELEMENTS OF BEHAVIORAL THEORY

After **Ivan Pavlov** discovered classical conditioning, wherein physical reactions can be evoked by manipulating the stimuli that trigger them (e.g., pairing food that made dogs salivate with ringing a bell, then fading the food until the dogs salivated upon hearing the bell alone), operant conditioning eventually followed. **Edward Thorndike** proposed the Law of Effect: any behavior followed by desirable consequences is likely to be repeated, while any behavior followed by undesirable consequences is likely to cease. An important difference between classical and operant conditioning is that the former involves reflexive actions, whereas the latter involves a choice by the individual. **John Watson** established the theory of behaviorism in the early 20th century, defining applied psychology as a purely objective experimental science aiming to predict and control behavior. His behaviorism was founded on the principle that only behaviors that can be externally observed and measured can be studied. Internal consciousness or emotions could not be observed by others; hence radical behaviorists found these could not be objectively studied, described, or quantified. **B. F. Skinner** is known for his work expanding and refining behaviorist theory, including the principles of behavior modification.

## TRANSACTIONAL STRESS-COPING MODEL

A stress-coping model is one used to evaluate stressors that affect an individual and the manner in which the individual copes with these stressors. Various models have been developed for specific populations, such as those with gambling addiction and those with schizophrenia. The *Transactional Model of Stress and Coping* (Lazarus and Folkman) can apply to multiple populations. This model states that stress may result from environmental (flood, war, disasters) or life events (divorce, illness, deaths). The individual responds to stress in a number of steps, but responses are mediated by the individual's personality, belief system, and relationships:

- **Cognitive appraisal**: Primary appraisal determines how significant the stressor is and secondary appraisal determines how the stressor can be controlled or coped with.
- **Coping strategies**: Includes problem-focused strategies to decrease stress and emotion-focused strategies to decrease the emotional response to stress.
- **Therapy**: CBT helps the individual to view situations in such a way as to reduce stress and improve the emotional response to stress.

## CARL ROGERS THEORY AND THERAPY TECHNIQUES

Rogers defined *unconditional positive regard* as treating others with acceptance and approval for who they are, regardless of what they do or any other limiting conditions. Rogers also named *conditions of worth* as the opposite of unconditional positive regard. He said parents making their love or approval conditional upon certain required behaviors by their children applied conditions of worth. Rogers found children treated thusly became adults whose self-esteem depended on others' approval instead of being innate affirmations of self. Rogers also advocated empathy. Experts advise TRSs that in counseling, they should convey empathy, not sympathy. Sympathy is feeling sorry for clients, undermining objectivity/clear judgment. Empathy is putting oneself in the client's place to understand the client's experience without becoming overly emotionally involved. Listening without responding—including silent listening and note-taking practiced by some traditional psychoanalysts—is passive. Active listening involves eye contact, postures, gestures/other indications of listener acceptance and response. Reflective listening restates listener perception of speaker messages for confirmation/correction, and/or states perceived feelings behind/implicit in messages.

## FLOW THEORY

Flow theory (Csikszentmihalyi) states that various mental states can help or hinder learning. Completing a task/learning requires both challenge and skill and a balance. If, for example, the challenge is low and the skill level is low, the client may feel apathy, but if the challenge is low and the skill is high, the client may feel relaxed. Flow occurs when both the skill level and the challenge level are high. Flow is the mental state most conducive to learning. Whether in work, play, recreation, or leisure activities, the client must be intrinsically motivated or gain some type of satisfaction and motivation from carrying out tasks designed by others. The characteristics of flow include:

- Having the ability to completely focus and concentrate on a task.
- Being clear about goals/rewards and feedback.
- Transforming time (seems to slow or speed up).
- Completing the task effortlessly.
- Finding a balance between challenge and skills.
- Merging actions and awareness.
- Feeling in control.

## THEORIES OF PLAY

Theories of play applied to TR/RT services include:

- According to **Surplus Energy theory**: After individuals have had their basic needs met, play results from their having remaining excess energy. Recreation theory states: When physical energy is overused, fatigue occurs, producing the need to play.
- **Pre-exercise theory** proposes: Inherited characteristics are the sources of an instinct for engaging in play.
- **Recapitulation theory** posits: Elements intrinsic to the development of the human race are recaptured through the process of play. Relaxation theory states: The need to relax is the motivation for play to occur.
- According to **Catharsis theory**: Children temporarily resolve conflicts/partly satisfy drives through play when other means are not available.
- **Compensatory theory** says: When the means of accomplishing one's goals or desires are blocked, play serves as an outlet which substitutes for those goals and desires.
- According to **Psychoanalytic theory:** Play serves wish-fulfillment needs; through repetition, addresses situations that provoke overwhelming anxiety, both adaptively and defensively; and helps gain control and mastery over threatening events.
- **Instinct-Practice theory** argues that play helps animals/humans survive by practicing and perfecting skills they will need as adults.

- From the perspective of **Developmental theory**: In each stage of cognitive development, children construct and shape their reality behaviors and their play behaviors. Young children demonstrate their development of the ability for symbolic representation when they engage in make-believe and pretend play.
- **Generalization theory** maintains: Participants can generalize any of the play behaviors that they have learned to other settings and applications.
- According to **Attribution theory:** An individual's locus of control primarily determines the forms of play in which the individual is engaging.
- **Achievement-Motivation theory** proposes: Play behavior demonstrates the desires of individuals to strive, succeed, and excel.
- According to **Optimal Arousal theory**: Elements of play include components that combine both novelty and complexity in order to engage and sustain the participants' attention and interest.
- From the viewpoint of **Conflict-Enculturation theory**: Play enables the participants to experience and learn new behaviors in safe environments.

## THEORETICAL PERSPECTIVES ON PLAY FROM THE 19TH AND 20TH CENTURIES

In the late 19th century, the public recreation movement advocated that organized recreation for all children be provided. The theoretical bases for this movement include the following concepts:

- **Play as a social necessity**: Joseph Lee, considered the father of the American play movement, furthered the establishment of many playgrounds and recreation centers. He helped the idea of play as an important child development and community life influence gain public acceptance. His contemporary, Luther Halsey Gulick, also viewed play as vital to community life.
- Wayne Stormann identified **play's utility** for coordinating body functions, promoting health, providing manual training, and preparing children for "indoor confinement" in school and then factory work.
- Progressive Era reformer Jane Addams, founder of Chicago's Hull House Settlement and winner of the Nobel Peace Prize, identified opportunities for organized play as **necessary antidotes to poverty for children**.
- **Self-Expression theory:** Physical educators Elmer Mitchell and Bernard Mason theorized that since human beings were dynamic and active, they needed outlets for energy, to express their personalities, and utilize their abilities.
- Mitchell and Mason identified anatomical and physiological structure, physical fitness levels, social and family backgrounds, and environmental factors influencing in which **kinds of play activities individuals engaged**.

## SOCIOLOGICAL DESCRIPTIONS OF PLAY TYPES AND STYLES

French sociologist Roger Caillois categorized **four types of play activity** across cultures:

- *Agon*: competitive games/activities
- *Alea*: games of chance
- *Mimicry*: make-believe/pretend play
- *Ilinx*: dizziness-inducing play (e.g., spinning/whirling, swings, seesaws, certain dances, roller coasters, bungee-jumping, skydiving)

He also identified two play behavior extremes:

- **Paidia**: spontaneous play
- **Ludus**: controlled play with rules

All four play types can be at either end/anywhere in between.

In *Homo Ludens (Man the Player),* Dutch social historian **Johan Huizinga** defined play as pervading life; voluntary, not required; beyond meeting physiological needs; separate in time and place from ordinary life; controlled by rules, demanding exact order; characterized by tension and uncertainty; and, while having an ethical value by requiring rule compliance, unconcerned with good/evil. Huizinga classified play activity into two types: contests for something and representations of something. He saw play as a significant civilizing influence in society, citing ancient Greek society's permeation with play forms.

## PSYCHOLOGICAL ASPECTS OF PLAY ACCORDING TO FREUD

Sigmund Freud found play therapeutic: Complex/confusing/unpleasant life circumstances often overwhelmed children, and they could re-experience and reinterpret them through play, gaining control over them. Freud saw play as children's way of coping with reality—playing with it, making it less threatening, more acceptable, and mastering it. He compared playing children to creative writers, creating their own worlds by rearranging elements of the real world in more pleasing ways; described children as taking play "very seriously", investing much emotion in it. He wrote, "The opposite of play is not what is serious but what is real." Erik Erikson, Anna Freud, and others influenced by Freud experimented with play therapy for troubled children. Child psychologist Lawrence Frank wrote that play is an important factor in children's psychological development, describing play as a way children learn things nobody can teach them. Through play, children orient themselves to and explore the environment of space, time, objects, structures, animals, and people. They learn symbolic meanings and values, delayed gratification, progressive striving, discovery and experimentation. Through play, children learn in unique, individualized ways. They continually practice subtle, complex communication and living patterns that adult social life will require them to master.

## IMPACT OF PLAY ON THE SOCIAL DEVELOPMENT OF CHILDREN

Many experts find that children's success in school is in large part dependent on their ability to interact positively with peers and adults. Play has a vital role in children's social development. Playing has the following social benefits for children:

- When they attempt to gain entry to play already going on, negotiate the roles involved in play with others, and learn to appreciate others' feelings while they are playing with them, children have many opportunities to practice both verbal and nonverbal communication skills.
- When children must wait for and take turns while playing organized games, share play materials and activities, and respond to their playmates' feelings, these experiences all help to develop children's social skills for interacting with others and their personal growth.
- When children play with others, they come into contact with the needs and wants of other people. This enables and directs them to experiment with the roles of others in their homes, schools, and communities.
- When children play with others, they must work out conflicts over rules, materials, and space in positive ways. Having to do so enables them to experience other people's points of view.

## RECREATION

Definitions of recreation in the professional TR/RT literature have included the following common elements:

- Recreation is activity, rather than rest or total idleness.
- Recreation includes a broad range of individual and group activities with single, episodic, or frequent and sustained lifetime engagement.
- Recreation is voluntary activity, rather than obligatory or compulsory.
- Recreation is motivated internally by desires to attain personal satisfaction, rather than motivated externally by imposed goals or rewards.
- Recreation is not identified by what individuals or groups are doing as much as their reason(s) for doing it. What defines an activity as recreation is the way the person feels about it. Recreation depends on the participant's attitude or state of mind.
- While recreation is usually primarily motivated by seeking pleasure, it can also fulfill physical, intellectual, or social needs. Recreation can offer trivial or light fun, serious self-discipline and commitment combined with reward and fulfillment in some cases, or frustration, or even pain in some cases.

### BENEFITS OF RECREATION

Recreation opportunities make communities healthier and stronger. People want to settle in desirable communities; parks and recreational facilities enhance community socioeconomic status, image, and desirability. Recreation promotes cleaner, safer neighborhoods, livelier community atmospheres, and brings neighbors together. When people retire, they want community recreational opportunities. Well-maintained parks and recreation facilities help decrease crime in surrounding urban communities: patron presence in and around facilities is an effective deterrent. Parks and recreation areas and opportunities also help youth avoid criminal activities, decreasing juvenile delinquency. After-school recreation programs reduce crimes against and by children. Lower crime rates increase resident security and property values. Recreation activities further volunteerism. People using parks and recreation facilities and programs are more willing to volunteer. Parks and recreation departments depend on volunteers for program and service delivery. Volunteer pride and dedication augment their interest and engagement in other community functions. Park and recreation participation develops stronger outdoor, natural resource, and environmental stewardship; unites families; promotes social bonds and cultural tolerance; supports seniors, child and youth development, and citizens with disabilities; enhances cultural diversity and harmony; enhances education; and prevents negative social behaviors like teen pregnancies and substance abuse.

### PSYCHOLOGICAL ASPECTS OF RECREATION

Research finds that regular physical activity through recreation can make many mental health disorders less severe, enabling improved coping with daily life. Not all mental health benefits of recreation even require physical activity. Physical activity, participation in hobbies, recreational activities with friends, and social interactions during park and recreation activities are found to reduce depression in all age groups. The relaxation, rest, and revitalization afforded by recreational activity relieves stress, psychological tensions, and anxiety. People find that being in pleasant outdoor settings, such as wilderness areas and natural spaces within urban areas, to be soothing and calming. Group recreational activities strengthen social connections among people. Self-image; self-esteem; personal growth; spiritual reflection and expression; and personal, neighborhood and community life satisfaction are benefits whereby participation in recreational activities enhances quality of life for people. Those who participate in recreation are found to be noticeably happier. The more often they engage in recreation, the more likely they are to be completely satisfied with their career choices, friends, and perceived life success. Research (ARC, 2000) finds significantly more people participating in outdoor recreation satisfied with personal health, fitness, and quality of life than those not participating.

## LEISURE

### THEORETICAL PERSPECTIVES ON LEISURE

(1) **Elite, aristocratic ancient Greeks**, not needing to work, viewed leisure as ideal freedom for intellectual enlightenment and activity. The ancient Greek word *skole/scole,* meaning leisure or a scholarly discussion place, is the root for Latin *scola/*English *school/scholar,* showing the Greeks' close relationship between leisure and education. (2) 19th-century sociologist **Thorstein Veblen** depicted leisure as emblematic of social class in *The Theory of the Leisure Class*—the "idle rich" upper class, needing not work, supported by lower-class labor. Increased working-class leisure, and many wealthy people's increased working careers, have since contradicted this view. (3) **Sociology**: leisure as discretionary/unobligated time free from work. A criticism is that intrinsically/extrinsically rewarding, obligated/unobligated activities can overlap in nature/characteristics. (4) **Social science**: leisure as physically active/passive activity during free time. While individual perceptions of activities as enjoyment or obligation can contradict this definition, TR/RT scholars like David Austin define leisure by intrinsic motivation/self-determination. (5) **Holistic lifestyle leisure** defined by perceived freedom; activities for their own sake in self-actualization. (6) Leisure as **uplifting, holy**, contributing to religious values/spiritual expression. (7) Leisure as **contributing to social capital** by enabling people to associate/interact/act collectively.

### CONCEPTS OF LEISURE THROUGHOUT THE LIFESPAN

What leisure consists of and how people pursue it continues to change throughout the lifespan. Leisure may be considered a privilege or a right. Given a definition of leisure as free time, adults who work frequently see leisure as a reward they earn for working, hence a privilege. Some working long hours with limited leisure time, which they find indispensable and precious, may regard it as a right. Working people might regard the leisure of people born into privilege as a gift. Leisure seen as a privilege is unequally distributed: only those qualifying obtain it as a reward. Depending on their circumstances, some people perceive it as having worked enough all week to earn days off on the weekend; others may qualify to purchase some types of leisure by having enough money. Theoretically, leisure seen as a right should be equally distributed. Most cultures believe humans have certain natural rights. The US defines inalienable human rights as life, liberty, and the pursuit of happiness. In the US, the natural right to the pursuit of happiness can be interpreted to include the right to leisure.

### SOCIAL BENEFITS OF LEISURE

Research shows family bonds and cohesion are strengthened by leisure activities. Family studies find positive correlations between family leisure engagement and family life satisfaction. 43% of Americans reported being introduced by their parents to their favorite leisure activity and 16% by other relatives (ARC, 2000). Most Americans consider family togetherness, and sharing and bonding over experiences with family and friends, important reasons for physical and outdoor leisure activities. Research regularly finds higher marital satisfaction in couples spending their leisure time together. Culturally diverse people are less concerned with their differences, and more with having fun, during leisure pursuits. Leisure activities enable sharing cultural and ethnic differences. Visiting cultural or historic sites, museums, fairs, festivals, and other outdoor cultural events are popular leisure activities: educating people about other cultures prevents misunderstandings/"clashes" among groups, contributing to society's overall functioning. Playing games erases social distinctions among participants; ability to play the game determines their status. Leisure arts programs improve participant attitudes about trust, other-acceptance, and self-expression. Leisure programs/activities offer more social opportunities for people with disabilities and senior citizens; prevent youth social problems; and develop child/youth cooperative behavior, social skills, decision-making, problem-solving, critical thinking, and conflict-resolution skills.

## SPECIAL POPULATIONS

### HOMELESS/LOW INCOME

TRS intervention with **homeless/poor clients** should be provided in client neighborhoods, be holistic and comprehensive, and collaborate with other practitioners. This includes referrals, parent and family education, training, consultations with criminal justice workers and psychiatrists, and facilitating access to funds and transportation as well as leisure experiences. TRSs must overcome obstacles for clients like drug dealer and gang presences, user fees they cannot afford, other participation requirements, facility locations, staff and other user attitudes, and media program publicity which clients cannot understand or access. Practitioners must combine empathy and nonjudgmental attitudes with setting expectations and enforcing rules. They can encourage clients to set realistic goals, consider the consequences of their actions, and make decisions by listening supportively without giving advice about problems without solutions or patronizing clients. They can help clients overcome disenfranchisement by offering them community responsibilities, engaging them in program delivery to enable control, self-determination, social support, interdependent functioning, and resource acquisition, making them feel similar to, not different from, peers. Integrating assertiveness training, time and stress management, and creative/expressive activities help clients dissipate frustration and anger, relieve tension, and cope better with everyday survival needs.

### INTERVENTIONS

For clients who are prison inmates, residents in mental health facilities, or living in VA medical center placements, TRSs include skills for activities of daily living in their treatment protocols, as well as gardening, operating coffee houses, and other activities that provide incentives. TR/RT interventions with socially disadvantaged children combine structured and unstructured activity to enable them to develop both academic support skills and playfulness. Physical activities, libraries, small-animal projects, gardening, and environmental education are among the programs they can offer to children. Clients living in homeless shelters can be assisted in coping with social decompensation through TR. TRSs can design programs that provide leisure and recreation activities while supplying positive role models, helping clients develop their social skills, and offering clients involvement in experiences that will foster networks and connections within their home and community environments. TRSs can also provide clients with empowerment for taking initiative and independent action through experiences to develop alternative leisure skills, self-care classes, grieving seminars, financial planning, travel planning, and developing and implementing personal leisure and life plans.

### INDIVIDUALS WITH DISABILITIES

According to research, approximately 40 million/12–20% of Americans have some kind of disability. Historically, they lacked access to many recreational and leisure activities, especially outdoors, because recreational facilities were built considering only nondisabled people, and no special equipment was available. Two major events/processes in recent history changed that:

- A number of nonprofit organizations were formed with missions of advocating for disabled people to enhance their quality of life. These groups' efforts include providing specially adapted equipment for recreational activities and offering opportunities to disabled people to engage in outdoor and indoor recreation they formerly could not access.

- When Congress enacted the Americans with Disabilities Act (ADA) of 1990, it guaranteed persons with disabilities the same fundamental civil rights as other disenfranchised groups had previously been afforded by constitutional amendments. The ADA mandated publicly used facilities to provide access to people with limited mobility. The federal government has since funded construction of hundreds of outdoor recreational facilities accessible to people using wheelchairs, walkers, crutches, canes, etc. Supported by the ADA, activists then started lobbying state and local agencies for increased opportunities, resulting in an exponential increase in outdoor recreational access for the disabled.

## DIVERSE LEISURE AND RECREATIONAL ACTIVITIES FOR UNIQUE CLIENTS

Today, numerous TR/RT activities suit a diverse range of clients. For example, the **Therapeutic Recreation Directory** lists nearly 500 ideas for TR treatments and activities. There are activities designed for use with people who have Alzheimer's disease, enabling participation with consideration for their symptoms of memory loss, confusion, and disorientation, and additional activities for people with other dementias. For people with physical disabilities, there is information for playing adapted badminton, adapted gardening, adapted wheelchair tennis, chair exercises, and even Tai Chi in chairs. For aging adults, activities like Hobo Party/Amusement Park Game emphasize the therapeutic power, cognitive memory stimulation, and pleasure of reminiscing. Activities like Bad Jokes of the Day use humor therapeutically. There are leisure awareness activities; activities with balls and balloons; water activities; racing activities; and social activities like card games, Bingo, cooking club, arts, crafts, etc. In addition to social activities, there are solitary activity ideas. Daily living skills and coping skills activities are included. Conversation groups and many other activities afford cognitive stimulation. Community service, outing planning, team-building, self-esteem, self-expression, and many more activities are available.

## CLIENTS WITH MENTAL ILLNESS

The **"Know Thy Neighbor" game** (TR Directory website) addresses the isolation, withdrawal, and inappropriate social interactions characteristic of mental disorders. Instead of the artificial setting of role-playing, or discussing them instead of practicing them, recreational activities provide a natural vehicle to **develop social skills**, with real-life opportunities for clients to use required skills and encounter the natural consequences of their behaviors. This game can be adapted for small and large groups. Its goal is for clients to get to know one another. The TRS writes 20 or more questions whereby clients can get information about other participants, and distributes these questions to them before or during the activity. The TRS divides the group into two teams. After reading the first question aloud, the TRS asks the second team to vote whether they believe more than half of the first team voted "Yes." If they guess correctly, they earn a point; if incorrectly, the first team gets the point. TRSs can stop and invite clients to tell stories some questions trigger for them. Ideas for questions include naming their favorite color, music, fast-food restaurant, and activity; whether they are superstitious; if they have ever experienced love at first sight, etc.

# Design Program Services

## PSYCHOLOGICAL BENEFITS OF LEISURE ACTIVITIES

People interviewed by researchers have reported that participating in leisure activities helped them to cope with major traumas like deaths in their families. People also report that leisure gives them an escape from everyday stressors. Studies have found positive correlations between participating in multiple leisure activities like visiting with friends, engaging in hobbies, and swimming, and decreases in participants' levels of depression. The more time people spent on leisure activities, the more their depression diminished. Other researchers have discovered that when people even recall outdoor leisure activities they have engaged in, their moods become more positive, raising their self-esteem and lowering their depression and rates of suicide. People experience personal growth through engaging in leisure activities. They can develop skills unrelated to their job skills and working lives, express themselves in ways they cannot at work, and affirm their identities. They can explore their sense of self and inner spiritual selves, forming new identities and new behaviors. Today, rather than identifying with their job titles, people are beginning more often to identify themselves by their leisure pursuits.

## LEISURE ACTIVITIES FOR CHILDREN FROM BIRTH UNTIL SCHOOL AGE

While some Americans may view leisure as a privilege for working, others view it as a right. The US Declaration of Independence asserts the human right to life, liberty, and the pursuit of happiness. One way people pursue happiness is through leisure activity; therefore, leisure can be considered a human right in America. In fact, the National Recreation and Park Association (NRPA) position statement on inclusion affirms the right to leisure as a necessary condition for human beings to ensure their wellbeing and dignity; part of a productive life and healthy lifestyle; something all individuals are entitled to for self-expression and pursuit, development, and improvement of abilities and talents in inclusive settings, wherein all possible opportunities, environments, settings, and skill levels should be offered.

**Children from 0–6 years** have rights to leisure as vital to their growth and development; children, unlike adults, need not earn leisure. Activities should have short durations corresponding with young children's attention spans and emphasize gross motor skill development through body awareness, large unstructured movements, and rhythm. Children at these ages are examples demonstrating the surplus energy theory: they typically need activity to expel abundant energy.

## LEISURE ACTIVITIES FOR CHILDREN AGES 6 TO 12 YEARS

Even though physical growth and development from **6–12 years** old are not as rapid or dramatic as from 0–6 years, they are still significant. Older children need physical activity, especially to enable normal bone growth and also to develop their strength, coordination, flexibility, and agility, as physical exercise is a continuing requirement for normal development. An additional dimension of leisure activity becoming more important during children's school-age years is their emotional and social development: their environment expands, they are exposed to more social interactions with peers and adults, more friendships, and many new academic challenges and activities. When their motor skills progress, children develop not only physical mastery, but also acceptance from peers and personal feelings of accomplishment. Leisure and recreation activities further children's individuality, independence, sensitivity to peer points of view, cooperative behavior, and socialization. Without real financial/employment responsibilities, and with ongoing developmental needs, older children have rights to leisure like younger children. Leisure activities for older children most demonstrate the surplus energy, stimulus arousal, instinct practice, and self-expression theories of play and leisure.

## LEISURE ACTIVITIES FOR ADOLESCENTS

**Adolescents** experience drastic, fast changes typical of puberty and many other significant life transitions. In their cognitive development, teenagers become more able to grasp and interact with abstract concepts. This changes their capacities for not only working with more intellectually advanced academic subject matter, but also considering their and others' emotions in more abstract and complex ways; appreciating social interactions and relationships more abstractly, with more complexity, sophistication, and delicacy; and understanding responsibilities at higher levels, enabling their assuming additional responsibilities as adults often expect of them. In terms of intellectual, adaptive, and social development needs, teens have rights to leisure to facilitate their development. Leisure also becomes a privilege as adults give them desired reinforcements for successfully fulfilling new responsibilities, undesired consequences for failing to do so. Adolescents can apply more advanced, complicated rules, strategy, reasoning, and interaction in sports, non-physical games, and other leisure activities.

## LEISURE ACTIVITIES FOR ADULTS

**Adulthood** comprises the majority of the lifespan. Adult leisure activity is less focused on developmental needs than with children, more on individual participation benefits. Since adults have more responsibilities with college, employment, serious intimate relationships, marriages, and families, leisure activities are less unplanned/spontaneous, more scheduled. For adults, leisure becomes less a right and more an earned privilege for working and meeting responsibilities. Adults are more frequently responsible for others, not just themselves. Thus, they more often engage in leisure benefiting their families, rather than pursuing only individual activities. Stimulus arousal theory applies to adult leisure as adults typically demand activities engaging and sustaining their interest. Relaxation theory applies more to adults than most children because after working hard for a living, adults have greater needs for relaxing and enjoying free time. The compensation and spillover theory applies most to adult leisure: some adults compensate for work by engaging in opposite/completely different leisure activities (e.g., engineers creating paintings); others have spillover leisure (e.g., writers doing crossword puzzles or composers attending concerts).

## LEISURE ACTIVITIES FOR OLDER ADULTS

Although retired **older individuals** typically have more leisure time, restrictions on their activity include chronic health problems/medical conditions, fewer peers due to mortality, greater social isolation and smaller support groups/networks, reduced finances, more limited living conditions, and greater needs for assistance from others for social contact and interaction. However, today people are also living and working longer and are healthier, better educated, and more active at older ages. Leisure activities can enhance older individuals' physical and mental health by improving, preventing, mitigating, minimizing, reducing, or reversing age-related conditions, including cholesterol, blood pressure, cardiovascular status, overweight, obesity, underweight, loss of muscle mass, loss of flexibility, blood sugar, type 2 diabetes, etc.; enhancing coping with age-related changes; improving balance, strength, coordination, endurance, functional independence, and cognitive functioning; and promoting feelings of competence, control, and confidence. Leisure activities/programs enable more frequent, regular social contact and interaction. Leisure education connects older people with social services networks, including medical care, transportation, health and nutrition advice, and financial management resources. Leisure involvement can also make life more meaningful for retired people.

### BENEFITS, BARRIERS, PREFERENCES, AND OPPORTUNITIES

TR experiences enhance wellbeing, health, and life satisfaction for **aging individuals** through the following:

- Promote functional independence
- Stimulate cognitive processes and continued learning
- Promote continuing contact with reality and current events
- Increase sense of competence, self-worth, confidence, and control
- Provide opportunities for social interaction, offsetting isolation and loneliness
- Enable adaptation to leisure time
- Enable meaningful contributions and roles
- Prolong interest and responsibility for their own wellbeing
- Help them adjust to losses and changes related to aging.

**Barriers to participating** include fear of falling, worry about physical and psychological safety, visual and/or hearing limitations, loss of family and friends, embarrassment about incontinence, impeded motivation due to dependence on others for transportation, inclement weather, etc. Aging adults would rather engage in leisure activities similar to what they previously enjoyed than "senior" activities they perceive as identifying them as old. Since aging is associated with decreasing exercise, physical activity lowers blood pressure, raises HDL (beneficial) cholesterol, stimulates the brain, decreases need for medications and doctor visits, motivates social interaction and active lifestyle, lowers risk of falling, eases self-care, motivates better nutrition and diet, and prevents age-related disease. Moreover, later adulthood affords opportunities to volunteer and otherwise apply amassed life experience, education, knowledge and learning.

## RELATIONSHIP BETWEEN LEISURE FUNCTION AND OTHER FUNCTIONAL DOMAINS

Models of TR/RT outcomes encompass domains of physical, mental, emotional, spiritual, and leisure functioning. While these all interact, **leisure functioning** is regarded as both distinctive from the others and highly related to them all. TR/RT outcomes can be envisioned as a combination of health status, ranging from death to optimal wellness, and functional potential or capacity, from minimum to maximum. Quality of life, manifested by self-reported/expressed qualities of self-determination, wellbeing, satisfaction, contentment, and joy, is seen as a function of both health status and functional capacity, increasing as they increase. TR/RT has specific leisure assessment instruments, included in comprehensive assessments informing TRSs of client needs for planning interventions to help improve, maintain, or regain overall functioning levels. TR/RT interventions include leisure experiences TRSs facilitate for clients. TRSs design intervention strategies that further leisure functioning, leisure independence, and leisure lifestyle among other outcomes. Leisure education is typically a component of comprehensive TR/RT programs. Work and play/intervention and leisure are dynamically interrelated: while performing difficult tasks, clients experience fun and enjoyment. Studies find enjoyable activities more effective for achieving long-term attitude and behavior changes, making this intervention-leisure interrelationship therapeutically ideal.

## SELECTING INTERVENTIONS
### RELATIONSHIP BETWEEN INTERVENTION AND LEISURE EXPERIENCE

One factor that influences how much emphasis is placed on either intervention or leisure experience in the nature of TR/RT services provided is the **philosophy** of a particular TR/RT agency or individual TRS. At one extreme, some may advocate an approach that focuses exclusively on client leisure experience; at the other, some may believe in focusing exclusively on intervention. The goals of the TRS/agency are another factor, related to client needs. For example, someone with an acute injury might have greater needs for intervention to achieve rehabilitation; people with chronic illnesses, workaholic adults living with too much stress and not enough fun, or abused children might have more need for the therapeutic effects of play. The setting where TR/RT occurs is another factor. Hospitals and rehabilitation centers involve more intense focus on diagnosis and treatment characteristic of acute-care approaches; home health care, day habilitation, and outpatient services have a more community-based focus on health promotion and education. Where TR/RT is found on the continuum of this service delivery model will affect how much emphasis is placed on leisure experiences vs. interventions.

### CORE LEISURE ACTIVITIES VS. BALANCE LEISURE ACTIVITIES

According to the core and balance model of leisure activities, **core leisure activities** tend to stay the same throughout life, whereas **balance leisure activities** change along with the changing needs of the individual and/or family. In family leisure, core activities are shared in common by family members and occur regularly, whereas balance leisure activities in families are planned and occur less frequently. Some examples in family leisure of core activities include family dinners, daily family prayers, and board games that families play together. Some examples of family balance leisure activities include going to movies, outings to the park, camping, and vacation trips. Core leisure activities provide structure, familiarity, and stability; balance leisure activities provide novelty, change, challenge, and variety. For families, both types of leisure activities promote cohesion through participating together; balance activities promote group and individual adaptability through challenging them to adjust to changes. Core activities are typically less expensive, less planned, more spontaneous, and shorter in duration. Balance activities are typically more expensive, require more planning, and last for longer times.

## USING RECREATION AS A TREATMENT MODALITY

Since the early days of the development of psychoanalysis, psychiatry, and psychotherapy, practitioners like Sigmund Freud and others influenced by him, including his daughter Anna Freud and psychosocial development pioneer Erik Erikson, experimented with play therapy as a way to alleviate children's emotional and psychological disturbances. Play therapy continues to be utilized today as a way of relieving stress, diverting attention from obsessive preoccupations, enabling children to express themselves, and teaching them alternative coping mechanisms and expanding their skill repertoires. Depression in adults and children often responds to recreation as a treatment: recreation involving physical activity is proven to elevate the mood and improve cognitive and physical functioning. Non-physical recreational activities also engage the mind, improve the mood, and afford social interaction. Recreational physical activities dissipate anxiety; non-physical recreational games, hobbies, and social interactions distract attentional focus off worrying and release tension. People with cognitive disabilities/injuries benefit by learning rules, applying strategies, and solving problems during recreational activities. Those with physical disabilities/injuries can regain, improve, and maintain strength, balance, coordination, flexibility, and endurance through targeted TR/RT activities.

## ASSERTIVENESS TRAINING

Many clients, including those with disabilities, abuse victims, and others with low self-esteem have difficulty expressing their emotions and preferences, requesting what they need/want, and standing up for themselves and others. **Assertiveness training** is an action-oriented, popular intervention addressing these issues. Through instruction, modeling, and role-playing, TRSs help clients learn to recognize feelings and overcome challenges to express them appropriately in workplaces, other social settings, and relationships. Honest communication demonstrating respect for self and others characterizes assertive behavior. Clients learn to examine and counter irrational beliefs impeding assertiveness, employ "I statements," and behave not passively or aggressively, but assertively. A related intervention is physical confidence therapy (PCT), which has been found helpful to adults and teens with low self-awareness, self-esteem, self-confidence, self-discipline, and impulse control. Small groups (4–6 members) meet for 45-minute sessions several times weekly. Each individual sets personal goals. TRSs lead them through progressively structured routines, basing movement to successive levels on member mastery according to high, TRS-defined standards. Group discussions of experiences incorporating open emotional expression are important. Clients actively participate in helping other group members.

## STRESS MANAGEMENT

Because the body, mind, and spirit are strongly interactive, research finds many debilitating effects on the body from protracted stress. Some studies reveal the majority of primary care physician visits are stress-related. Technological advances, while affording many new leisure opportunities, can also replace physical activity with sedentary choices. Physical leisure activities improve health status, including helping to manage stress. Depression is the most common mental health problem experienced by Americans today, and **stress management techniques** that include complying with CDC physical activity recommendations are found to relieve depressive symptoms. People with disabilities often lack access to and resources for managing stress; TRSs can help by providing programs including stress management activities, helping clients locate and access resources for continued management, and teaching them techniques/activities they can practice at home. Many TRSs and other therapists use biofeedback, yoga, therapeutic massage, aromatherapy, meditation, and other relaxation techniques in various settings, as treatment approaches congruent with current holistic disease prevention and health promotion models. Recent research also supports humor therapy, including movies, recordings, books, and games, for managing stress.

## SOCIAL SKILLS TRAINING

Leisure behavior frequently requires social interaction skills, which may be the main reasons for some leisure activities or their effects. Many individuals with disabilities are often identified as lacking sufficient social interactions skills, requiring direct instruction to remediate these deficits, and being at risk for future life functioning if they are not remediated. **Social skills training** has the goal of developing clients' fundamental interpersonal and social skills they require for functioning in society. Therapists teach clients appropriate nonverbal and verbal communication techniques for responding in various social situations. Clients practice maintaining eye contact, carrying on conversations, responding to instructions, interacting appropriately with the opposite sex, and other social skills. Training frequently includes modeling, role-playing exercises, video feedback, and real-life practice homework. Studies find various people with and without disabilities benefit from social skills training, including individuals with physical impairments, developmental disabilities, severe disabilities, mental illnesses, substance abuse disorders, and behavior disorders; children with learning disabilities; aging adults; prison inmates; and people at risk of incarceration. By teaching expected social behaviors, social skills training prevents/remediates social isolation and rejection and enhances self-esteem, self-control, awareness of others' rights, and social inclusion.

## COMMUNITY REINTEGRATION

**Community reintegration** entails resuming clients' typical behaviors, activities, and roles that have been interrupted by injury, illness, and/or disability. These include productive behaviors, activities with families and social contacts in natural community environments, and independent and interdependent decision-making and problem-solving behaviors. Clients who have encountered medical and/or behavioral health issues are assisted in returning to their communities by community reintegration interventions, which are integral components of rehabilitation programs and complete therapy cycles. Skilled nursing, rehabilitation, outpatient, home health, and community TR/RT services incorporate community reintegration. Community reintegration is included in care plans for clients who have had strokes, head injuries, spinal cord injuries, chronic pain conditions, mental health disorders, and substance abuse disorders. Interventions used in community reintegration include leisure assessments, leisure education, leisure counseling, leisure resource guidance, socialization with non-disabled peers, peer mentoring, fitness activities, developing functional individual and family recreation skills, time management, stress management, and problem-solving skills training. Managed care restrictions shortening inpatient stays and resulting recidivism are addressed by community reintegration experiences, which also comply with the national public health agenda focusing on secondary condition prevention and health promotion for persons with disabilities.

## BEHAVIOR MANAGEMENT

Behavior management and modification are frequently used in TR/RT programs because they have the advantages of being effective with clients regardless of their intellectual, cognitive, emotional, and social levels and status, and they work to change only behaviors that are outwardly observable and measurable, regardless of client inability to communicate inner feelings and thoughts. One example **is aversion therapy.** To help clients stop smoking, drinking, overeating, abusing substances, etc., behavior modification pairs the stimulus to which the client is attached with unpleasant stimuli, rendering it less desirable. Another example is **cognitive restructuring**, which shows the client some behaviors are founded on irrational assumptions and replaces them with more adaptive beliefs and behaviors. Albert Ellis's Rational-Emotive Behavior Therapy, a form of cognitive-behavioral therapy, makes extensive use of this technique by identifying unrealistic, negative beliefs and self-talk and reteaching more logical concepts and positive self-talk. An additional behavioral technique is **contingency contracting**. The therapist writes a contract, which the client agrees to, stating which consequences are contingent on specified undesired behaviors, and which reinforcements/rewards are contingent on desired behaviors. Behavior contracts are useful with children having behavior disorders and others having social and rule compliance issues.

### REINFORCEMENT

In behaviorism, **reinforcement** means anything immediately following a behavior that the individual finds rewarding, increasing the probability of the individual's repeating the behavior. Punishment is anything immediately following a behavior that the individual finds aversive, decreasing the probability of repetition. When a behavior's function is to get attention, withholding attention eventually extinguishes the behavior. **Positive reinforcement** presents something rewarding; positive punishment presents something aversive. **Negative reinforcement** removes something aversive, not presenting anything; for example, telling a child he or she can skip a hated chore like taking out garbage for completing homework. Schedules of reinforcement can be continuous or partial; ratio or interval; and fixed or variable. Individuals often come to expect reinforcement on fixed schedules, only responding accordingly, or become satiated and stop responding. Hence intermittent reinforcement, which is unpredictable, is more powerful and resistant to extinction.

**Partial reinforcement** produces slower, but more extinction-resistant learning than continuous reinforcement. **Fixed-ratio reinforcement** schedules cause steady, high response rates, with short pauses after reinforcement. **Variable-ratio schedules**, which are unpredictable, produce steady, high response rates, as in gambling. **Fixed-interval schedules** create high response rates late in the interval, but slower rates right after reinforcement. **Variable-interval schedules**, which reinforce after unpredictable lengths of time following responses, cause steady, slow response rates.

### PREMACK PRINCIPLE

The **Premack principle** states that pairing an undesirable stimulus with a desirable/reinforcing stimulus makes the undesirable thing more reinforcing/desirable. This is applied in behavior modification to increase preference/decrease aversion. For example, a child who hates broccoli but loves cheese may be enticed to eat broccoli by serving it with cheese sauce. Successive approximations are used in shaping: individuals receive rewards reinforcing responses progressively closer to ultimate desired responses. For example, agoraphobia is treated by first rewarding stepping outside the door; then walking some distance; then visiting a lightly populated place, then a slightly busier location, etc. Time-out briefly eliminates reinforcement by removing someone to a neutral reinforcement-free location; this produces extinction of attention-seeking/reward-seeking behaviors.

## MODALITIES AND FACILITATION TECHNIQUES TO APPLY TO PROGRAM DESIGN

To help clients attain specific therapy goals they have identified together, TRSs choose certain activities that will restore or improve client functioning related to those goals. They also choose certain **facilitation techniques** that will have the most positive impact on the client's health status, function, and quality of life. These techniques are based on research findings documenting their effectiveness with particular client populations. These achieve better, more predictable results for clients and also ensure higher accountability and quality for health insurance providers and regulatory agencies. Because insurance companies increasingly limit terms of care due to escalating hospital costs, TRSs must design brief treatments that are effective enough in shorter times. This includes not only designing new interventions, but also TRSs reevaluating their own functions and roles and modifying treatment goals and adapting intervention strategies so they fit into the time/session limits imposed by benefits coverage, are congruent with their agencies' goals and treatment approaches, and also meet the clients' needs and goals.

## ACTIVITY MODIFICATIONS

TRSs and other staff can adapt to continually changing work conditions, accomplish more in less time with fewer resources, and plan experiences for maximal client benefit by examining and interpreting the TRSs' activity and task analyses. Some experts recommend approaching programming creatively and, before making changes, considering the nature of a client's activity participation. Adaptations TRSs can make include securing, changing, or making equipment; altering the method(s) the client uses for performing a task; and changing the procedures or rules to compensate for certain required skills. Adaptations to equipment include: changing the color of material, changing surface texture, reducing noise, changing equipment weight/size, subtracting/adding equipment, controlling light and temperature. Adaptations to methods: decreasing the number of steps in a task, decreasing the number of facts to remember, decreasing the number of objects to manipulate, choosing from fewer alternatives, offering fewer/more choices. Adaptations to procedures/rules: permitting less/more time, adjusting scoring, changing number of positions, adjusting area size, changing distances, adding rest intervals, changing number of participants, eliminating winning/losing.

### MODIFICATIONS FOR PARTICIPANTS WITH DISABILITIES

To enable **maximum participation in leisure and recreation activities** for clients with disabilities, the first choice is modifying the activity, not eliminating it or substituting a completely different one. One way to modify activities is changing the equipment. For example, badminton can use a yarn ball or a balloon, which clients can strike with racquets more easily, instead of a shuttlecock/birdie. In other adaptive badminton games, TRSs may substitute foam "lollipop" paddles for racquets. The paddles are lighter in weight, easier to manipulate, and less likely to injure others. When modifying activities, the activity should stay as close as possible to its original form. Another way to modify activities is changing the rules of the game/sport/activity. Some examples involve playing tennis, badminton, basketball, and other sports/games in wheelchairs. Ball-handling/racquet-handling rules must be changed, as participants also use their arms and hands to propel/maneuver wheelchairs (e.g., wheelchair tennis rules allow players to let the ball bounce twice if necessary, and only the first bounce must be within bounds).

### ADAPTIVE RECREATION

For persons with disabling injuries, illnesses, or conditions, TR/RT processes, techniques, equipment, and other **factors must be adapted or modified** for the specific impairment to enable the participation of the particular individual. Adaptations are based on client strengths, avoiding interference with their impairments while allowing them to demonstrate their skills. They are of a temporary nature, individualized, and can change as the client's abilities progress and impairments recede. TRSs planning interventions and transitions with clients and caregivers consult resources for support in providing adaptations that empower clients and enhance their performance. A noticeable example of an adaptation is the use of a wheelchair for ambulating during sports events. A less obvious one involves longer times for resting during sports competitions. Additional examples include preferential seating/positioning for vision and hearing impairments; Braille, large print, and magnifiers for visual impairments; adaptive mechanical devices for impaired movement and control; slowing, shortening, simplifying, and repeating instructions/activities for intellectual disabilities; shortening instruction and activity durations for AD/HD; and eliminating/controlling various environmental stimuli for autism spectrum disorders.

## TYPES OF ADAPTIVE DEVICES

**Adaptive devices** cover a wide range, from simple tools to mechanical apparatus to sophisticated technological items. Individuals with impaired/limited fine motor skills can use eating utensils with larger handles/adapted grips. Before the advent of sophisticated electronics, persons who temporarily/permanently lost arm/hand use could write via a simple mechanism clamped to a desk/table, holding a pencil/pen they manipulated with their mouths. Some people lacking functional manual grasp have eaten more independently using feeding machines, on which they pressed knobs rotating a plate and operating an arm that scooped with and extended a spoon. The greater height and enclosure of Carrington walkers provide body support for walking upright. People who cannot ambulate on foot can use wheelchairs. With rehabilitation and training, some amputees graduate from wheelchairs to walking and even running on prosthetic limbs. Patients recovering from injuries or illnesses can progress from wheelchairs to walkers, then quad canes, then single-point canes—indefinitely or on the way to walking unaided. Individuals with severe cerebral palsy/other conditions causing paralysis participate in aquatics activities sitting in the sling-like Hoyer lift, which raises/lowers/laterally moves them for short distances. This device also helps caregivers with transfers, bathing, and other ADLs.

## ASSISTIVE TECHNOLOGY

Efficacy research studies have found that **computerized TR/RT programs and leisure education programs** are effective for enabling youth with intellectual, psychological, and behavioral disorders to acquire social skills knowledge. These programs have the advantage of being interactive, engaging participants, and affording the opportunity to learn autonomously at their own paces, increasing independence, self-awareness, self-regulation, control, and self-esteem. They also free much valuable TRS time for hands-on therapy and supplement TRS instruction. Individuals having difficulty with social interactions can learn more easily, including social skills knowledge to enhance future interactions. Virtual reality activities allow client participation in widely varied simulations, enabling desensitization to fear of heights and other phobias in safe environments, relaxation in soothing/pleasant environments, etc. Computer games not only provide leisure activities, they also include games providing leisure education. People can locate accessible community facilities/activities online. In physical rehabilitation programs, physical functioning, attention, memory, recall, and cognitive reintegration are enhanced through Wii Fit and other computer games. Seniors and children gain communication and social interaction through Skype and online networks. Research predicts computer literacy and internet use can counter age-related declines, prolong independence, and improve leisure and quality of life.

### IMPACT OF ASSISTIVE TECHNOLOGY ON INDIVIDUALS WITH DISABILITIES

Researchers into the use of assistive technology by individuals with various disabilities have reported these people gained greater physical wellbeing, independence, better functioning in ADLs, and more access to self-determined leisure and social opportunities. Wheelchairs and other adaptive devices enable access to transportation, education, and employment; **adaptive toys** provide children more leisure options. One population especially benefiting from assistive technology has severe/profound multiple developmental disabilities and/or communication disorders. Studies with microswitch-based equipment and programs have found participants demonstrated enhanced moods and manipulation responses. In one individual example, a young wheelchair-bound woman with profound intellectual disability, hearing impairment, and diplegia enjoyed watching TV, but had no control over it. A residential facility professional procured her an adaptive remote control with very large buttons, placed on her wheelchair's lap tray. With the palm of one hand she could turn the TV on, off, change channels, and adjust the volume. This freed staff from TV duties; eliminated her dependence on them for this leisure activity; reduced boredom and frustration; and afforded her greater control, choice, autonomy, enjoyment, and a significant leisure asset for her transition to community living.

## TYPES OF ASSISTIVE TECHNOLOGY FOR CHILDREN WITH SPECIFIC DISABILITIES/IMPAIRMENTS

Many assistive devices that help students in school also help them in TR/RT. Children with attentional, memory, vision, reading, and/or processing deficits can use audio recorders and players to capture speech, to supplement text they have to read or replace it, and to repeat instructions they cannot attend to or remember the first time, reducing TRS work. These are also useful for home practice. Children with AD/HD, ASDs, or cognitive disabilities benefit from timers—hourglasses, wristwatches, etc.—to address pacing/timing problems and help them transition from one task to another. For leisure activities involving reading, plastic reading guides help with focusing and visual tracking problems. Children who have attentional deficits and sensory processing issues can use inflatable seat cushions to provide stimulation and movement, helping them focus their attention without needing to stand up and walk around during seated activities (relaxation exercises, listening, discussion groups, verbal games, board games, arts & crafts, etc.). FM listening systems help children with hearing impairment, auditory/language processing disorders, ASDs, and AD/HD by amplifying speech and minimizing background noise. Graphic organizers are valuable low-tech aids for organization and memory problems.

## ACTIVITY ANALYSIS

When planning a TR/RT program for a client, the TRS first identifies which specific experiences will best enable the client's accomplishing measurable results by analyzing each stated client objective and finding all content that can promote this accomplishment. Then the TRS identifies the most effective leadership approaches and interaction techniques for working with the client when implementing the TR/RT program. To effect desired changes in client skills and behaviors, the TRS selects the most appropriate content, modifies it as needed, and sequences it correctly using **activity analysis and task analysis**. Activity analysis is taking a particular leisure experience and identifying every physical, cognitive, psychological, social, and spiritual behavior involved. The TRS determines why a certain leisure experience will likely help ensure the best therapeutic benefits through the activity analysis process. Task analysis is the process of ordering each of the component skills performed in an activity, listing each individual skill identified during the activity analysis. Every step in the task represents a measurable outcome; the TRS establishes objectives for each step and monitors progress toward them. Through skill sequencing, the TRS can start intervention at the client's ability level and identify client skill mastery for meeting objectives.

## EVALUATING CLIENT PROGRESS USING ACTIVITY ANALYSIS

Since the TRS originally conducted an **activity analysis and task analysis** for identifying which content and strategies to select to enable the client to attain the goals/results defined, the TRS will also use these tools for modifying leadership strategies and adapting program content as needed. When the TRS realizes that the client will probably not achieve desired results using the originally planned intervention content and strategies, he or she re-interprets the initial activity and task analysis findings to adapt program content. The TRS might then have the client utilize different skills, less complex skills, or more advanced skills for making the experience successful. For instance, the TRS could re-analyze the sequence of skills, and then begin the therapy with a different step in that sequence. He or she might also change the resources and/or procedures used to make the therapeutic activities less or more difficult/challenging as indicated. In modifying/adapting programs, TRSs may also incorporate caregiver and team member ideas and resources based on their observations of the client in other settings.

## USING THE ACTIVITY ANALYSIS TO INFORM A TASK ANALYSIS

Before conducting a task analysis, the TRS completes an **activity analysis**. Through the activity analysis, the TRS identifies every component behavior of a specified leisure activity, categorizing them into physical, cognitive, psychological, social, and spiritual domains to identify which leisure experiences will be most effective in helping the client attain goals and objectives identified in the individual therapy program plan. The activity analysis informs the ensuing task analysis: The component behaviors identified in the activity analysis designate each individual skill the client needs to perform the activity. The TRS lists these skills in the order of performance. Breaking the task down into sequential steps represents task analysis. Each step is designated a measurable outcome, for which the TRS writes an objective. During therapy, the TRS monitors client progress toward these objectives. As an example, a client whose mobility was recently impaired must learn to ambulate using a wheelchair. Task analysis **steps** would include: (1) Transfer from bed/chair to wheelchair. (2) Maintain sitting balance. (3) Grasp and release the seat belt. (4) Grasp and release wheelchair brakes. (5) Propel the wheelchair forward, backward, and turn it. (6) Stop the wheelchair.

## DOMAINS ASSESSED DURING THE ACTIVITY ANALYSIS

During activity analysis, TRSs identify every behavior a client must perform during a selected leisure activity. These behaviors are categorized into physical, cognitive, psychological, social, and spiritual domains of experience. Activity analysis allows TRSs to discern which experiences will best help the client attain the goals and objectives identified for him or her and why these activities will be most effective. For example, suppose a client's discharge goal is to live in a transitional program, with a long-term goal of participating with significant others in community reintegration activities and short-term goals of identifying accessible community leisure programs, developing community safety and travel skills, and developing leisure skills compatible with significant others' leisure skills/activities. Corresponding objectives are stated in measurable terms. An accompanying activity analysis could include: Physical—grasping and releasing, extending and flexing the elbow(s), strength, endurance, stamina, and sitting balance. Cognitive—remembering criteria for accessible parking areas, understanding accessible travel routes to enter buildings. Psychological—listening and responding to/interacting with others. Social—identifying one's own and others' leisure preferences, discussing leisure likes and dislikes. Spiritual—accepting adaptations, valuing leisure's benefits.

## CHAINING

**Task analysis** consists of breaking down a given task into its smallest parts or steps, to learn in the same order as they will be performed. Learning one step at a time facilitates successfully acquiring complex, multi-step skills for persons with disabilities and makes learning new tasks easier for everyone. TRSs/other professionals instruct the individual in one step until mastered. The TRS then teaches the second step. Before proceeding, the TRS then has the client learn to connect the first and second steps. This process is repeated with each step, adding one more consecutive step, and once mastered, learning to perform the first, second, third, etc., steps in a row. The behavior modification technique of chaining is similar to task analysis by guiding the individual through a series of tasks, beginning with the simplest skill to progressively more complex ones. Forward chaining is essentially the same as task analysis in teaching the first step until mastered, then the second, etc. Backward chaining begins with the last step in a sequence, proceeds to the next-to-last step, and continues until the first step is reached.

## APPLYING A TASK ANALYSIS TO TEACHING SKILLS TO CLIENTS WITH DISABILITIES

Clients with intellectual, cognitive, behavioral, sensory, and other disabilities have difficulty performing complex tasks containing series of actions because they cannot attend to, remember, and/or learn all actions simultaneously. Many of us take for granted being able to perform tasks with multiple components. This is partially due to our ability to pay attention to, consider, process, understand, and acquire a number of parts within the whole at once. However, it is also partially due to our having learned everyday tasks to the point of automaticity: we are no longer conscious of the individual steps involved. If we think back, though, we remember when we first learned to tie a shoelace, ride a bicycle, or drive a car, we had to learn the new task performing one step at a time and then combining steps into the whole sequence. People with disabilities are the same, except they often need smaller, shorter steps; simpler instructions; longer times; and more repetition and practice to master tasks. **Task analysis benefits** them by breaking a task down into brief, concrete, manageable steps, learned one at a time.

# Implementation

## Deliver Program Services

### INDIVIDUAL VS. COMPREHENSIVE PROGRAM PLANS

TR/RT program designs at the **individual and comprehensive/agency levels** have many similarities. Both follow the APIE sequence of assessment, planning, implementation, and evaluation. A TRS may integrate several individual clients' individual program plans into existing agency programs and/or develop new programs to meet the needs of all clients accessing the agency's services or programs. Whereas individual assessment collects client baseline data, comprehensive assessment uses those data to determine whether each client is integrated into existing programs, or new programs must be designed to meet his or her needs. TRSs organize programs reflecting ranges of client characteristics like assessed skill levels, needs, health status, leisure behaviors and preferences, and content areas or inclusive services according to diagnoses, before designing a comprehensive program's vision, mission, purpose, and goals. They also consider future environments and settings to which clients will transition. Influences on comprehensive programs include professional, government, and regulatory standards; department/agency documents; department/agency service scope; funding, resource, facility, equipment, supply, and staff availability; written department/agency plans of operation; and professional research literature reviews regarding treatment efficacy.

### ACTIVITIES FOR SENSORY STIMULATION

One very simple **sensory activity** that TRSs report clients find amazingly enjoyable is giving them bubble wrap and letting them pop the bubbles. Not just children, but adults with Alzheimer's disease and other dementias absolutely love this activity, which provides stress management as well as sensory (tactile and auditory) stimulation. Many adults without impairments also love popping bubble wrap. An activity that stimulates each sense while affording relaxation, a calming environment, and a sense of wellbeing for a small (3–6 people) group is to bring a box containing the following items: a binder filled with pictures, a Lava Lamp, and a glitter ball for visual stimulation. For tactile stimulation, the glitter ball, a textured ball, PlayDoh, and a shower puff. A diffuser with essential oil/lavender-scented shower/bath gel/body wash stimulates smell. In some facilities, fire codes prohibit diffusers: put body wash in a bowl and run hot water over it. A CD/MP3 player with relaxation music stimulates hearing. Any edible/drinkable/tasteable items client diets permit stimulate taste and serve as refreshments. Place items on a table; bring clients into the room, encouraging them to explore items and express any memories/stories stimulated by pictures/fragrances/tastes, etc.

### FACILITATING THERAPY PROGRAMS FOR SPECIFIC CLIENTELE

#### CLIENTS WITH DISABILITIES

When implementing TR/RT programs with clients who have **learning disabilities, behavior disorders, motor skills disorders and/or communication disorders,** TRSs should define the expectations, boundaries, rewards, and consequences in advance to afford safe, positive environments. Their interventions, supervision, and follow-through should be immediate and firm to promote appropriate client behavior and compliance. TRSs should design programs that emphasize self-esteem, self-regulation, self-initiation of behaviors, development and application of problem-solving skills, and the formation of social relationships. TRSs can incorporate training in negotiation, conflict resolution, and instruction in how to give and accept criticism and praise to develop client social skills during training in recreational and physical activity. To help clients learn

117

motor sequences, socially appropriate behaviors, impulsivity moderation, and conflict resolution, TRSs can employ strategies like modeling, role-playing, and positive self-talk. They can develop client self-awareness, other-awareness, coping skills, and role expectations through techniques including relaxation, assertion, animal-assisted therapy, videotaping, and challenge/adventure courses.

### CLIENTS WITH OSTEOPOROSIS, ARTHRITIS, OR SPINA BIFIDA

TRSs help clients with **osteoporosis** and paralysis slow calcium loss rates by designing passive ROM exercise programs; help ambulatory osteoporosis clients by designing programs including resistance and weight-bearing exercises (e.g., yoga, walking); and, through YMCAs/other community agencies and outpatient clinics, design and administer programs for preventing falls. TRSs design programs for **arthritis** patients preventing joint trauma by avoiding fall risks, contact sports, gross motor activities, and weight-bearing exercises. Program designs incorporate ROM exercises, swimming, cycling, stretching, horseshoes/other throwing/target games, creative movement; relaxation exercises; anti-inflammatory and steroid medications; heat applications; bed rest; and avoidance of weight-bearing or sitting for long times. Program design for **spina bifida patients** includes promoting postural alignment; upper torso strengthening; weight management; and prevention of secondary contractures, pressure sores, and skin lesions. Exercises include ROM exercises; strength training; archery; swimming; chair aerobics; integrative sports, recreation, and play experiences to promote social interactions and friendships; and assistance with adapting to the energy output required for using mobility aids to ambulate.

### CLIENTS WITH OSTEOGENESIS IMPERFECTA, AMPUTATIONS, OR POLIO

Clients with **osteogenesis imperfecta (OI)** have brittle bones, so TRSs design programs wherein environmental barriers are minimized and clients learn to avoid and/or adapt to them, to minimize fracture risks. As they sustain fewer fractures, OI patients can begin to participate more in social interactions, swimming, ROM exercises, and wheelchair activities including competitive sports for some individuals. A program design consideration for **amputees** is that they are less active physically as a group. Therefore, TRSs design programs promoting physically active lifestyles, with rehabilitation goals and activities including ROM exercises and improvement, strength training, energy conservation, endurance training, residual limb care, correct body alignment, activity adaptations, and participation in community recreation. For clients who had **poliomyelitis** and may demonstrate the group of sequelae known as **post-polio syndrome**, TRSs apply caution regarding requirements for strenuous physical activity, particularly since gauging the extent of impairment and lesion levels is difficult because polio paralysis is incomplete. In program planning for this population, TRSs include temperature variation control during activities, formal wellness classes, and support group activities to promote high-protein, healthy diets, and teach activity level self-monitoring for participating in community recreation.

### CLIENTS WITH ORTHOPEDIC IMPAIRMENTS OR BURN INJURIES

**Orthopedic problems** include injuries and chronic disorders. Orthopedic treatments include casting, bracing, and surgery. Activities that require bearing weight for protracted durations, or applying direct force to an involved joint, are contraindications for clients with orthopedic conditions. For these clients, TRSs design TR/RT programs to strengthen and stretch involved muscle groups, promote wheelchair sports, and include aquatic exercise. TRSs provide creative expression activities as emotional outlets and to help clients with lifetime impairments adapt.

**Burns and other thermal injuries** often disfigure patients, sometimes necessitating surgical reconstruction. Thermal injuries, their rehabilitation, and pressure garments often worn, limit mobility. TRSs design programs incorporating bedside activities to distract attention from debridement and skin grafting pain; ROM exercises; and relaxation training to develop coping skills for protracted splinting and bracing. Deformities change client self-images and others' reactions: TRSs include family and friends in programs. They use phased community reintegration for client preparation. TRSs encourage physical activity to enhance physical wellbeing and appetite. Unaffected skin sweats more to compensate for scar tissue lacking sweat glands: TRSs are alert to the dangers of dehydration and heat stroke.

### CLIENTS WITH ALZHEIMER'S DISEASE AND/OR DEMENTIA

TRSs can access the **Memory Programs** website, www.MemoryPrograms.com, to use Memory Programs with 1–20+ clients. They need only a DVD player and remote control. Memory Programs are TV activity games that engage clients with dementia; facilitate reading for people with visual impairments; encourage clients to interact socially about the programs; and additionally help individuals with "sundowning" symptoms to calm down. Staff members at long-term care and assisted living facilities using Memory Programs have reported that patients with dementia display more positive behaviors and wander less and that nursing staff experience more productive environments. Independent living communities have also expressed interest in Memory Programs and request their staff to use them at least once weekly. In Shopping Scavenger Hunt, TRSs list items for 1–20 participants to search for and cut out of newspaper sale ads; whoever finds the most wins. This activity helps Alzheimer's patients learn what things cost today—about which most typically have no idea—while having fun. Even low-functioning patients can participate; higher-functioning patients can search for the lowest/highest-priced items. Cutouts can be saved for a later collage activity.

### CLIENTS WITH MULTIPLE SCLEROSIS, CEREBRAL PALSY, OR SEIZURE DISORDERS

TRSs must consider **MS** causes thermal sensitivity/heat intolerance: aquatic activities should be in cool (80–83°), not warm (84–88°) water. Otherwise, aquatic therapy can help manage MS symptoms and afford enjoyment. To prevent contractures and promote relaxation in MS and CP patients, regular stretching exercises help. TRSs must monitor exercise levels to prevent fatigue. Medications prescribed for MS often cause transient shortness of breath, flu-like symptoms, and depression, impeding performance and causing discomfort; TRSs need familiarity with these. Clients with **seizure activity** must have partners and close supervision during horseback riding, swimming, rappelling, and similar activities. TRSs must also document durations and types of seizures to help medical staff examine the relationships among seizure symptoms, drug therapies, and activity levels. TRSs must additionally monitor medication side effects impeding social and physical behaviors. By helping clients and others consider how their perceptions regarding seizures affect social interactions, TRSs promote psychological wellbeing. When helping **CP** patients transfer to/from wheelchairs, TRSs must understand abnormal reflexes affecting movement and accordingly adjust handling techniques. CP clients with spasticity find continuous movements easier; those with athetosis find intermittent movements easier. Breathing exercises, sports, and music remediate CP client visual, communication, and perceptual deficits.

### CLIENTS WITH CANCER

Clients with **life-threatening diseases** such as **cancer**, and their families, need help not only with physical impairments, but also psychological sequelae like fear of recurrence, pain, and death; isolation; depression; and grieving. TRSs offer expressive therapies and journaling to manage frustration and anger and, after losses alter client self-images, help redefine self-concepts. Muscle relaxation exercises and guided imagery help decrease/manage anxiety and stress. Client spiritual health is enhanced through outdoor/nature experiences. Leisure education and group processes help clients make realistic choices, adapt their lifestyles, learn alternative coping skills and strategies, and develop their problem-solving skills. Medical play alleviates fear of cancer treatment in children and families. Youth with cancer benefit from adventure/challenge experiences with better health-related quality of life, self-esteem, and improved physical and psychological outcomes. Sadness is counteracted with therapy using humor. Client attention is diverted from self and illness through animal-assisted therapy, which fosters care of others. TRSs promote exercise, nutrition, and other lifestyle practices through social experiences and behavioral interventions, reducing risks for comorbid conditions like diabetes and cardiovascular disease. Physical activity and wellness programs support client physical wellness while focusing entire family units on quality of life.

## CLIENTS WITH MULTIPLE DISABILITIES

To help individuals with **severe multiple disabilities** choose and practice self-reinforcing experiences, TRSs consciously offer alternatives reflecting client preferences. Behavioral backward chaining builds independence/self-reinforcement. To improve skill learning/remediation and transfer and generalization to other tasks/situations/settings, TRSs include lead-up and follow-up strategies; practice in actual environments of skill application; and focus interventions on developing functional skills. To promote developing age-appropriate skills as well as generalizing skills and social inclusion, TRSs give clients training in leisure experiences they will use with future peers. Skill maintenance and transfer also improve through travel, money management, social greetings, and similar functional skills training. TRSs use individual observations to evaluate client progress because deficits/delays in one area can obscure gains in another: severe multiple disabilities' cumulative effects are interactive. Following environmental and preference assessments, TRSs more effectively respond to diverse individual client needs through 1:1/structured small-group interactions. Relaxation techniques like tapping/rubbing/massaging muscle groups opposite contracted body parts reduce muscular tension. Reactive recreation equipment (switches, remote controls, etc.) are naturally reinforcing, deliver sensory feedback and increase engagement and interaction. TRSs use prompts and cues in least-to-most intrusive sequence, from verbal to physical, and fade these, promoting self-directed behaviors, when equipment facilitates interactions.

## CLIENTS WITH HIV/AIDS

Teenagers and children with **HIV/AIDS** need to continue progress toward developmental milestones: TRSs include age-appropriate experiences promoting family recreation and developing functional skills. Youth participating in camping and adventure/challenge experiences get social approval, emotional support, and risk experiences, building self-concepts and peer relationships and combating depression and loneliness. TRSs include financial concerns in planning: adults are often unemployed, children/teens can be orphaned, caregiver support may be absent/limited. Support groups relieve client/caregiver financial/other stresses, also affording TRSs observation opportunities of caregiver-client dynamics informing intervention. Autonomous activities such as free weights, aquatics, or exercise classes enable participation as health allows, plus immediate self-assessment. Client participation in activity planning, implementation, volunteer opportunities, and leisure education fosters self-control, empowerment, and choice expression. TRSs offer experiences to fill unused time, relieve stress, and develop new social networks. TRSs determine youth motivations for substance abuse, other risk behaviors, and leisure preferences through self-awareness assessment and values clarification. They establish environments of unconditional positive regard, incorporating creative and social experiences affording humor and disinhibition, fostering satisfaction and happiness. Since fatigue worsens HIV/AIDS, TRSs monitor physical tolerance while providing aerobic and progressive resistance exercises enhancing cardiopulmonary and psychological health. Animal-assisted and horticultural therapies promote senses of life, growth, and love.

> **Review Video: AIDS Infections and Malignancies**
> Visit mometrix.com/academy and enter code: 319526

## CLIENTS WITH PSYCHOLOGICAL DISORDERS

TRSs give directions and explanations to clients in calm, consistent, matter-of-fact ways. Before interactions, they define and clarify their expectations, desired results, and acceptable and unacceptable behaviors, including their reasons and consequences. When clients attain desired goals, TRSs immediately acknowledge and reinforce this. They emphasize cooperation, not competition, in their interventions and avoid "winner/loser" labels. To support clients in staying engaged with reality and assuming responsibility, TRSs provide written information and instructions. They state information in positive terms ("Do this") instead of negative terms ("Do not do this"). TRSs confront common client defense mechanisms while continuing to provide positive reinforcement for all desired behaviors and attempts. They encourage clients to express frustration and anger verbally, and offer them various options to choose from for expression. They deliberately ignore client behaviors that cause no harm, particularly attention-seeking behaviors. Because building trust takes time, TRSs model desirable behaviors for clients and plan interventions to afford progressively greater degrees of self-expression and social competence within group contexts. TRSs are continually aware of environmental elements that can make experiences unsafe or create stress. They document any unusual client statements or behaviors.

## CHILDREN OR ADULTS WHO HAVE BEEN ABUSED

**Abused children/teens** find outdoor recreation safe in contrast to indoor environments where family have abused them. TRSs providing outdoor adventure activities follow with formalized debriefing, establishing atmospheres enhancing self-esteem, sharing emotions, cooperative and problem-solving behaviors, and expressive arts helping younger children interpret thoughts/feelings. At-risk youth/families benefit from educational programs including physical activity, assertiveness, values clarification, journaling, stress and time management, and relaxation, promoting coping with continuing stress, reducing risk behaviors. Adventure experiences with youth/families in residential treatment centers further healthy family dynamics. Abuse causes self-devaluation; clients overcompensate through attention-seeking behaviors, impulse-control deficits, overachieving, over-competitiveness, and "poor loser" reactions. Recognizing underlying motivations, TRSs redirect energy to realistic goals and acknowledging self-improvement through esteem-building interventions. Children/teens exposed to family violence often lack play/recreation friends and are hyper-vigilant. TRSs use play therapy and gradual transitions from small-group to larger-group cooperative activities. Leisure education including values clarification, goal-setting, social skills training, and choices enable client values affirmation, social relationships, and ability-appropriate activity choices. TRSs observe and report signs of abuse; provide consistent expectations, routines, structure, active listening, and reinforcement for psychological wellness, respite care for safety, experiential activities (e.g., animal-assisted therapy), creative and expressive arts, and physical activity, alleviating tension, affording opportunities to assess abuse-induced developmental delays.

## LEISURE EDUCATION

Leisure activities prevent boredom in all ages, delinquency in min-ors, deterioration in the aging, and contribute to quality of life. People encounter financial, temporal, health, social, cultural, experiential, and other barriers to leisure participation. People with disabilities especially experience leisure barriers due to complex daily living function challenges. TRSs help clients acquire knowledge, decision-making skills, and attitudes for optimum leisure function, typically including program components developing psychomotor, cognitive, and affective skills fundamental to engaging in different social and recreational experiences; leisure opportunity awareness; appreciation and understanding of leisure's role in improving quality of life; opportunities for exploring and experiencing various health-enhancing social and leisure experiences that promote appropriate leisure behaviors; and provide supplies, equipment, etc., enabling access. Studies show **leisure education** improves appropriate expression and independence across settings and populations including abuse victims, trauma survivors, individuals with developmental and physical disabilities, aging adults, and prison inmates. Benefits include longer, more frequent leisure participation and improved quality of life, self-determination, self-esteem, problem-solving skills, decision-making skills, personal competence, locus of control, and perceived freedom. TRSs often use values clarification identifying, defining, and/or developing personal value systems guiding behavior to eliminate attitude barriers to leisure participation and satisfaction.

## BENEFIT TO CLIENTS WITH VISION OR HEARING IMPAIRMENTS

In addition to helping clients with **vision and hearing impairments** develop the skills for and access participation in competitive sports events that are designed taking these sensory deficits into account, TRSs also help them adapt to different sports and achieve integration into community-based sports programs. They also offer leisure education programs that introduce blind/visually impaired clients to magnifying devices, the Optacon (optical to tactile converter), books with large print published by the American Printing House for the Blind, Braille books, etc., to encourage them to initiate self-directed leisure experiences. Moreover, TRSs help our growing population of aging citizens, which includes more members with visual impairments, to continue/increase social engagement and develop home-based activities through leisure education. Hearing impairment is also more prevalent in the aging population. TRSs use leisure education to help clients with deafness or hearing impairment to participate in leisure and recreational opportunities through leisure education, which promotes more positive attitudes and better social outcomes and decreases obstacles to participating.

## BENEFIT TO CLIENTS WITH MUSCULAR DYSTROPHY OR ARTHRITIS

Children and adults with **muscular dystrophy** have to adjust spending long periods of time in bed rest and sitting in wheelchairs. TRSs can provide leisure education that will help them adjust to these changes by developing their skills for and interests in leisure activities in which they can participate. These activities include writing in journals; using the internet to join and interact with support groups; activating TVs, toys, and other appliances that are equipped with remote controls by using light-touch equipment; expressing themselves through painting, drawing, soft sculpture, and other forms of art work; and playing cognitive games engaging their attention and interest without taxing them physically. People with arthritis also need to adjust to changes in their physical movement and leisure participation. Through leisure education, TRSs can help them adapt to such changes in lifestyle, comply regularly with routine physical activity, adhere to weight management practices to minimize stress on their joints, learn new leisure skills in which their participation is not restricted, and make them aware of inclusive options for wellness.

## BENEFIT TO CLIENTS WITH CHRONIC FATIGUE SYNDROME

The cause of **chronic fatigue syndrome** is unknown, and its course is unpredictable. Symptom relief and improvement of wellbeing and functional capacities are treatment foci. TRSs provide leisure education to clients through both individualized sessions and support groups. They promote information access regarding workplace and home coping strategies and support groups, and help them develop coping strategies, increase acceptance of the condition, and decrease anxiety. TRSs teach clients both to balance their physical activity and appreciate that despite their intense fatigue, which can discourage them from exercising, regular appropriate exercise actually affords numerous benefits. TRSs cultivate client engagement in social interactions and activities, offering support and minimizing depression and isolation secondary to their diagnosis. They introduce clients to the benefits of, and instruct them in, journaling and other passive leisure activities. Leisure education helps clients choose alternative experiences, monitor their daily activity routines, establish priorities, and realign goals. TRSs also help clients enhance their self-efficacy, personal control, and self-worth through leisure education by teaching them to focus on the present and improve their perceived quality of life.

## BENEFITS TO OLDER ADULTS

Leisure education with **older adults** helps them make choices, making them more likely to participate, be physically active, and practice lifelong sports and/or hobbies. Aging adults' motivations for self-directed leisure participation include spiritual wellbeing through meaningful commitments and contributions to others, satisfaction, cognitive stimulation, adventure, physical wellbeing, health, and companionship. Leisure education provides information and skills for such autonomous pursuits. Studies find leisure education contributes to life satisfaction by promoting feelings of independence and personal competence. It exposes seniors to social services resources for medical care, health and nutrition advice, money management, transportation, etc.; enables more positive perspectives, promoting resiliency from losses and more independent functioning; empowers decision-making regarding alternatives for spending time; identifies unmet needs, available resources, assets; and reinforces the importance of participation. In adult day care, respite care, in-home programs, and support groups, leisure education is essential to alleviate caregiver social isolation, reduced life satisfaction, and harmful effects of living without leisure. Leisure education improves senior brain fitness. Community stroke support groups use leisure education formats to promote resource awareness, social contacts, adaptations/modifications to prior leisure interests, health, and wellbeing for patients, caregivers, and families.

## LEISURE COUNSELING VS. LEISURE EDUCATION

**Leisure education** enables TR/RT clients to gain knowledge and develop decision-making skills and attitudes needed for ideal leisure functioning. This includes developing client psychomotor, cognitive, and affective skills for participating in leisure experiences/activities. Cognitive skills can include developing abilities to explore and identify personal leisure preferences and aptitudes. Leisure education also includes providing information, such as how and where to locate community leisure resources and facilities, including those accessible to people with various disabilities. Whereas leisure education concentrates on curriculum/program content needed for leisure engagement, **leisure counseling** entails personal development more than educational information. TRSs use specialized therapeutic and counseling skills proven instrumental for changing behaviors, attitudes, and/or thinking. Hence, when a TRS helps a client to eliminate personal barriers that interfere with leisure experiences, this process is more correctly termed leisure counseling than leisure education. As examples, TRSs might use behavior modification to eliminate/reduce agoraphobia impeding community leisure participation; or rational-emotive behavior therapy/similar cognitive-behavioral therapies to replace irrational/misleading thoughts impeding specific leisure behaviors ("I can't dance"/"I'm not strong enough to lift weights") or attitudes impeding general leisure behaviors ("hard workers don't have time for leisure"/"leisure is slacking off/self-indulgent").

## BARRIERS TO PARTICIPATION IN RECREATION
### ATTITUDINAL BARRIERS

TR/RT experts point out that the term "accessibility" means more than just physical accessibility, even though physical accessibility has presented major **barriers** to people with disabilities from participating in recreational activities and programs. For example, for people without physical disabilities who suffer from social impairments such as poverty and homelessness, requirements for participating in recreation can present barriers. Financial requirements/fees to participate in recreational programs, activities, and facilities represent particular obstacles for the poor. The location of a facility becomes an obstacle when it is not within walking distance of people's homes or jobs and people do not have and/or cannot afford access to transportation. Even when socially disadvantaged people can get to recreation facilities, they often encounter barriers in the form of the staff's attitudes toward them. Users with homes and/or more money may disapprove of their presence, and/or they may feel intimidated by them. Some recreational facility/program staff may not be culturally sensitive. Additional barriers to participation include gang presence and/or drug dealers in low-income neighborhoods.

## ARCHITECTURAL AND TRANSPORTATION BARRIERS

**Architectural barriers** can include stairs without ramps or elevators for people using wheelchairs, crutches, walkers, etc.; inadequate lighting and/or overly bright, glaring lighting for people with visual impairments; lack of Braille on elevator signs and other building signs, overly small signs, or no signs; building support columns, kiosks, platforms, and other objects interrupting open spaces that are difficult to navigate around for people with visual impairments and orientation and mobility issues; environments with high background noise levels for people with hearing loss; uneven flooring for people with balance problems and those using wheelchairs, walkers, crutches, canes, etc.; buildings with only audio fire alarms but no strobe lights for deaf people; inadequately amplified or overly amplified public address systems for the hard of hearing in buildings; fire and emergency exits not designed for/permitting access by people with disabilities; and many others. **Transportation barriers** include no available buses/public conveyances equipped with wheelchair lifts; train/rail stations with many steps and no or nonfunctioning escalators; no or insufficient elevators; lack of ramps in transit stations; airports with no or nonfunctioning escalators, moving walkways, etc.; lack of transit stations located near enough to some neighborhoods.

## ENVIRONMENTAL BARRIERS

People with disabilities can feel intimidated, even at agencies and organizations that offer welcoming atmospheres and the highest quality of inclusive service practices. They face **environmental barriers** including attitudinal barriers such as public misperceptions; architectural barriers such as obstacles and surfaces preventing them from navigating buildings and outdoor areas; ecological barriers such as mountains, trees, bodies of water, poor air quality, exhaust fumes and other air pollutants; transportation barriers; and economic barriers. In addition, state, local, organization, facility, or building rules and regulations that interfere with the access of people with disabilities to recreation services, activities, programs, and facilities constitute barriers. TRSs serve as resources to help individuals with disabilities and their parents and family members to overcome environmental barriers as well as personal intrinsic barriers that individuals with disabilities and their families experience to participating in recreation.

### OVERCOMING BARRIERS

There are several **considerations** to make for overcoming barriers to participating in leisure activities by persons with disabilities. Parents and caregivers of individuals with disabilities may have concerns that their children/family members lack the comprehension and/or skills to identify when they have free time; identify what they prefer or enjoy doing to have fun; know how to select, initiate, and participate in leisure activities; or are able to appropriately handle play materials and/or appropriately play with peers. Individuals with disabilities encounter both many environmental barriers and also intrinsic barriers caused by their own physical, cognitive, or emotional limitations. Intrinsic barriers can additionally include overprotective parents, educational and recreational segregation from peers, or lack of educational and recreational opportunities. Individual barriers are presented by lack of knowledge, social skills deficits, health problems, physical and psychological dependencies, and gaps in skills or challenges. Even when individuals can cope with internal barriers, they may still encounter environmental barriers including mountains, trees, and architectural obstructions. Nonphysical environmental barriers can include personal financial limitations, economic conditions, and negative attitudes on the part of the individual and/or of others.

# Adhere to Risk Management Protocols

## RISK MANAGEMENT PURPOSE AND ACTIVITIES

The development of procedures and processes for regulating delivery of safe, high-quality services is called **risk management**. Similar to quality improvement programs, risk and safety management aim to develop, monitor, and evaluate procedures such that operations are continually improved while clients and providers both remain unharmed. Because of natural and manmade disasters, catastrophic diseases, and terrorist actions, risk and safety management protocols have become integral parts of shared human experience, reflecting safety concerns on global as well as personal levels. Furthermore, as professionals, TRSs take part in activities that are designed for minimizing risk and loss and for promoting security and safety in workplace environments. TRSs are legally required to "act with reasonable care and prudence to prevent unreasonable risks of harm to participants" (Kaiser & Robinson, 2005). Personal or property harm due to failure to act reasonably and prudently, or due to one's actions, constitutes negligence. Four elements establishing negligence are: duty—identified TRS obligations to clients; standard of care—responsibility for providing the same care another competent TRS in one's position would provide; proximate cause—determining the TRS's action/inaction directly caused injury; and injury—an injury exists.

## LEGAL REQUIREMENTS FOR RISK MANAGEMENT

By law, TRSs must prevent unreasonable risk of harm to their clients by acting with reasonable prudence and care. Harm to persons or property incurred through professionals' failure to act thus, or through their actions, is defined as **negligence**. Establishing negligence requires four components: injury, proximate cause, standard of care, and duty. There must be injury for negligence to exist. Proximate cause refers to proving that the TRS's inaction or action directly caused the injury. Standard of care means the responsibility of the TRS to provide the same care that any other competent TRS would provide in the same position. Duty is the obligation to clients of the TRS, as defined in the job description, supervisory plan, or protocol of job duties and procedures. In planning and implementing risk/safety management programs, managers:

- Identify potential risk areas.
- Analyze the causes, severity, and frequency of incidents.
- Educate employees, interns, and volunteers regarding the implications and results of risk/safety management procedures.
- Implement plans for monitoring and evaluating services designed to prevent and correct safety risk behaviors.

## POTENTIAL SAFETY RISKS IN TR/RT PRACTICE

**Areas in TR/RT of potential safety risk** include: staff skills for lifting/transferring nonambulatory clients; staff-to-client ratios; programming issues (adapting and sequencing activities according to client abilities); client management issues (complying with requests, first aid requirements, and client elopement); and areas reflecting the primary role of communication in safety violations (medical charts, consent forms, or transactions revealing personally identifiable health information that could compromise client rights). After identifying and analyzing safety risks, managers may develop measures to minimize risk. TRSs can find risk/safety management policies in operations manuals. The Joint Commission, CARF International, other regulatory agencies, professional organizations' ethical codes, and standards of practice define safety practices. Risk and safety factors are covered in the ADA and similar laws. The Department of Homeland Security, other federal agencies, and local health departments dictate safety standards. Standard protocols often require first-aid training plus activity-specific credentials. Employers may require/provide professional liability insurance.

## MAINTAINING RECREATIONAL AND ACTIVITY AREAS FOR SAFETY

As part of the risk management policies and safety programs of hospitals and other facilities where they work, TRSs are typically responsible for **maintaining recreational and activity areas** and scheduling their use by patients/clients. These may include gymnasiums, weight rooms, picnic shelters, arts and crafts rooms, and TR/RT kitchens. To maintain safe environments within facilities, TRSs are responsible for locking activity and exercise rooms/areas and supervising patients/clients in these areas at all times. They are responsible to ensure that participants always wear athletic shoes in gymnasiums rather than street shoes, boots, sandals, or bare feet. If any equipment breaks, patients/clients/staff are directed to report this to TR/RT or maintenance staff. TRSs are responsible for limiting how many activities take place at the same time in gymnasium areas. They are also expected to identify all safety concerns and inherent risks associated with every activity and area to all participants. They must ensure participants wear goggles, smocks, gloves, etc., as each activity requires, and stringently control participant use of toxic and sharp materials. Making sure participants engaged in kitchen activities wash hands; keep tools, surfaces, and foods clean; and comply with dietary standards defined in facility P&Ps are other TRS duties.

## CLIENT INVOLVEMENT IN SAFETY AND EMERGENCY PRACTICES

By ensuring that TRSs, other professional staff, and clients are involved in **routine emergency and safety experiences**, agencies and service programs generate support of their security and safety policies and practices and exemplify this support, and make sure that staff and clients are prepared for emergencies and security and safety threats as well. The increasing cultural diversity of American communities includes growing numbers of residents with impaired mobility, older ages, and associated impairments. This makes it vital for TRSs to advocate for inclusive preparations for security, safety, and risk prevention and management, and to pursue continuing education and training in these areas. CARF International, the Joint Commission, and other professional organizations and regulatory agencies define risk and safety management practices in their ethical codes and standards of practice. Operations manuals, the ADA, the Department of Homeland Security and other national agencies, and local health departments also set standards for safety.

## RISK FACTORS AND SAFETY CONCERNS WHEN USING GYMNASIUM FACILITIES

TRSs are responsible for alerting **gymnasium** users to inherent risks in the facility and every individual activity pursued there. For example, in facilities containing floor carpeting, they must warn participants against sliding or diving after balls to avoid rug burns. They must alert participants if rugs conceal concrete floors, which can cause injuries from diving, flipping, tumbling, etc. TRSs/staff should provide mats for tumbling/other activities. In some facilities, wall padding can double as floor mats. Facilities without soundproofing can become very noisy, irritating AD/HD, anger management deficits, ASDs, and concentration difficulties. TRSs should advise participants before activities to self-monitor their reactions and practice self-control. TRSs should warn participants if gymnasium walls are close to play areas. Inherent risks in volleyball nets include cutting fingers/hands on the net and severe hand injuries from rapid crank unwinding if using the net crank without its safety latch. In addition to teaching weight users correct equipment use and requiring spotters, TRSs should inform them of safety hazards associated with weight room equipment, including others standing too near free weight users, others standing too near lateral weight bar users, and weights not having pins in place completely.

## MINIMIZING PARTICIPANT INJURY IN GYMNASIUM FACILITIES

Before high-intensity activities or game play, TRSs lead participants in appropriate warm-up activities like jogging/stretching/warm-up games related to main activities. Before every activity, TRSs teach participants required skills to ensure adequate competence, preventing pain/injury; encourage participant alertness, responsibility for their and others' safety; alert them to inherent activity risks; and review gym/activity hazards and safe behaviors. They strongly caution spectator alertness to avoid being struck by stray balls/objects. TRSs enforce storage/placement of equipment/clothes/other objects, preventing participant tripping. When leading activities, TRSs require suitable shoes and clothing, and jewelry removal before contact sports. TRSs watch for excessively aggressive play by stronger and/or more skilled players, since skill levels are often mixed, and direct such players to ease off with less able participants. TRSs set limits for multiple activities (e.g., tumbling, badminton, soccer ball kicking practice, and a basketball game should not all occur simultaneously within one gym). To avert elopement, major injuries, and assaults in hospital/psychiatric facility/prison gyms, TRSs must supervise every area used and be positioned to observe all activities. Soft-safe volleyballs, foam softball bats, and softer softballs reduce hand injuries indoors. Additionally, good judgment and common sense are imperative.

# Evaluation and Documentation

## Document Client Progress

### METHODS OF DOCUMENTATION

Various methods of documentation can be used in conjunction with one another or in isolation to assist the TR/RT process:

- The **flow chart format** and technique of clinical documentation are compatible with clinical critical pathway structures. A TRS using the flow chart method would document services and programs by the sequence in time whereby the client will be delivered each service. According to this planned sequence of intervention, the TRS would then document client responses and results.
- **Charting by exception (CBE)** is a method of only charting findings that are significant, or that deviate from professional protocols, standards, or clinical pathways. Variances are positive or negative: when expected results are different or delayed, they represent negative variance. When outcomes are accomplished sooner than expected, or are significant, these represent positive variance.
- Some hospitals use **source-oriented documentation** methods, wherein each patient's chart is divided into sections according to each professional discipline working with the patient. Each practitioner records all narrative notes on patient progress toward identified results in the section designated for that discipline. When programs are offered by human service and recreation agencies emphasizing education and health promotion more than treatment, TRSs keep attendance reports, activity protocols, observation logs, and anecdotal records.
- **Problem-oriented medical records (POMR)** organize client documents by problems/behaviors. Client charts are divided into five sections: data base, problem list, plans, progress notes, and discharge summary. Priorities are assigned to each problem. Professionals make chart entries not by their disciplines, but by problem areas.
- In the narrative part of the treatment plan, documents are organized according to the **SOAP notes method:** Subjective, Objective, Assessment, and Plan.
- Focus charting, similarly to SOAP notes, organizes the narrative section of a focus note by **DARP:** Data, Action, Response, and Plan. A TRS using focus charting would identify client concerns or behaviors and document an assessment, an implemented client experience, or other specific service component by organizing it into the four DARP categories.
- Also similar to SOAP and DARP is **PIE charting**: Problem, Intervention, and Evaluation. In PIE charting, the TRS would combine objective and subjective data to produce a problem list and document the interventions addressing the problems identified and the results of evaluations.

### SOAP NOTES

#### HISTORY

**Physician Lawrence Weed, MD**, first came up with the idea behind **SOAP notes in the 1970s.** He referred to it as the Problem-Oriented Medical Record, or POMR. Before this innovation, healthcare practitioners did not have any objective method for documenting medical records. As a consequence, physicians often made unscientific decisions about how to treat patients because they could not refer to records from other practitioners recorded in any systematic, organized manner. This caused a significant communication gap among healthcare providers. It was difficult to access

128

necessary charts; communication was unstructured; patient medical histories were not objective or consistently organized. This gave providers less control over patient care. As physicians adopted the POMR methodology, they came to name it SOAP, representing the four sections into which it divides medical charting: Subjective description, Objective measurements, Assessment diagnoses, and Plans for patient treatment. SOAP notes introduced structure and rigor to medical practice and a standardized system for communication among practices. Practitioners adopting the SOAP notes system in the early 1970s could retrieve and understand all records on a given medical problem for one patient. Today, electronic medical records systems are based on the original SOAP note principles and improve on its advantages.

## DESCRIPTION AND EXAMPLES

SOAP stands for **Subjective, Objective, Assessment, and Plan**. Healthcare providers frequently use SOAP notes as a method of documenting patient charts.

- The **Subjective** section typically includes the patient's presenting complaint and describes current patient condition in narrative form. It includes the onset of illness/injury and, if applicable, mechanism of injury; chronology since onset—worse, better, constant/variable/ episodic; quality of pain—sharp, dull, etc.; pain severity, usually from 1–10; factors that make the complaint better/worse—body postures/ positions, medications, activities, etc.; additional, significant symptoms related/unrelated to main complaint; other providers/treatments.
- **Objective** includes measurements like age, weight, etc.; vital signs; laboratory test results; physical examination findings.
- **Assessment** gives physicians' medical diagnoses made on the date of the note.
- **Plan** describes intended provider treatment actions (e.g., referrals, lab tests, procedures, medication prescriptions).

For example, a subjective SOAP note entry might be: "I found the patient on the floor next to his bed." A related objective statement: "The patient fell out of bed." A related assessment statement: "X-ray following patient fall shows right hip fracture." A related plan statement: "All shifts ensure bedrails are raised and locked; give patient emergency assistance; monitor levels of medication causing dizziness."

> **Review Video: How to Make SOAP Notes**
> Visit mometrix.com/academy and enter code: 543158

## DOCUMENTING COMMUNICATION

Clients, caregivers, and colleagues are more motivated and committed to the TR/RT process, and client assets are better utilized toward goal achievement, when TRSs communicate, share knowledge, and collaborate with them to avoid misunderstandings, minimize conflicts of opinion, facilitate mutual awareness of needs and assets, and ensure consistent service delivery. Collaboration in the development and implementation of service plans is also demanded by professional practice standards. **TRSs and all other team members document** their assessment data, goals, objectives, recommended intervention strategies, and therapeutic experiences in client individual program plans (IPPs), charts, and/or files. Through such documentation, TRSs inform and edify others regarding the purposes and nature of TR/RT services and programs. Team meetings, staff meetings, department meetings, and caregiver conferences include discussions of documented plans. For example, if team members learn from a client that family are not available for community activities, they must enlist friends/co-workers/acquaintances for meeting a long-term goal to participate in outings with significant others. If team and client concur that relaxation training and stress management interventions would be beneficial, they can add these to the IPP. Well-timed TRS invitations and sensitive responses encourage client participation, promoting self-determination.

## DOCUMENTING PROGRAM EFFECTIVENESS

Once TRSs have evaluated the results for their clients of their TR/RT programs, they report these during staff meetings with team members, clients, and caregivers; team meetings; and/or conferences. They use electronic files or forms their agencies have specified in their protocols or procedural formats. It is not unusual for a TRS to be assigned responsibility to keep records not only on a certain number of clients, but also a given number of programs. In this case, the TRS will not only report about measures of client results, but additionally document information about management of physical resources, financial management, management of staff, and similar component variables of the TR/RT program. For example, the TRS could write notes on client progress and record the results of evaluations conducted during TR/RT sessions and in addition, fill out monthly reports about inventory of supplies, expenses for specific events, income received, hours worked by part-time personnel, hours worked by volunteers, etc. By collecting and recording such data as these, TRSs provide information whereby agencies can evaluate the extent to which program management is supporting client results and also measure how effective the program is.

## DOCUMENTING AND ANALYZING CLIENT OUTCOMES

A TRS collects and records data on **client outcomes** to be accountable not only to agency management and regulatory and accreditation agencies, but moreover to the clients. TRSs use these data as quality indices and for analyzing program efficacy. Client satisfaction, and striving to meet client expectations through continually monitoring functions of staffing and use of resources, are emphases of quality improvement processes. To ascertain whether the experiences provided by a TRS are most suitable for assuring the client's outcome measures are attained, quality assurance audits are performed. TRSs also study outcome data from multiple clients in order to evaluate the effectiveness of their services and programs. This systematic collection of data to investigate benefits to clients and service effectiveness is called efficacy research. It shows how useful specific interventions are for meeting clients' specific needs. TRSs utilize user satisfaction surveys they administer to clients, and conduct case studies of individual clients, to report results for efficacy research and quality improvement programs when they are involved in these.

## USING DOCUMENTATION TO MONITOR CLIENT PROGRESS

**Monitoring client progress** toward attaining specified program objectives has primary importance because progress monitoring helps assure that the client reaches the therapy's short-term, long-term, and discharge goals. The TRS should document the content he or she has selected for the program, the facilitation techniques and modalities employed, the leadership strategies applied, how resources are managed relative to client objectives and potential, and how suitable these are. TRSs should also constantly consider whether alternative resources, experiences, and techniques could achieve the desired results more efficiently and effectively, and whether clients and caregivers are satisfied. Because unexpected reactions and results are as vital to the TR/RT process as the outcomes intended, TRSs should also document attitudes the clients express; how clients, caregivers, team members, and others react to the programs; and interpersonal and social interactions they observe during therapy. They can capture spontaneous responses through interviews and observations in leisure/recreation settings, and reviews of videos, photos, and completed projects. These help TRSs understand why clients do/do not attain objectives. Applying these methods helps clients and caregivers understand TR/RT and how it contributes to client wellbeing, change, and growth.

## Monitoring Progress for Transition or Discharge

In rehabilitation settings, the most frequently used assessment instrument is the FIM (Functional Independence Measure). TRSs can use the FIM to determine at which of **seven levels** a client initially functions in 18 areas of daily living activities, from completely independent at the highest level down to being unable to perform an activity at the lowest. Each level in between represents progressively greater amounts of assistance that the client needs to perform each activity. During rehabilitation interventions, the client's degree of disability will typically decrease and the degree of functional performance will increase in some or all areas. The TRS can re-evaluate the client's functional performance periodically during rehabilitation treatment using the FIM to document the client's progress over time. To help plan a client's discharge or transition to another program, the TRS can use FIM scores to predict how much assistance a client will need at home and what quality of life and life satisfaction the client might expect.

### Requirements for Discharge or Transition

Requirements that qualify a therapeutic recreation client for **discharge or transition** include:

- The client has completed the program as outlined on the client's treatment plan and achieved the goals and objectives.
- The client has shown a persistent lack of interest in the program and shows little interest in participation and has not, therefore, received adequate value from the program.
- The client must take medical leave to deal with physical or mental health issues and is not able to further participate in the program.
- The client has completed the medical treatment program and is no longer eligible for coverage for the therapeutic recreation program.
- The client refuses to cooperate or to participate in activities at all, so continued participation cannot be justified.
- The client signs himself/herself out of the program on own volition because of a desire to stop participation.
- The client's insurance carrier will no longer cover the costs of therapy, the client cannot pay privately, and no funding is available.
- The client has a need for a different level or type of service.
- Outline the elements of a discharge plan.

### Elements of a Discharge Plan

The elements of a **discharge plan** for a therapeutic recreation client may vary from one organization to another but generally include:

- Identifying information about the program and the client (name, birthdate, dates of admission and discharge).
- Diagnosis and rehabilitation problem list.
- Goals and objectives.
- List of all interventions utilized (includes sports, arts and crafts, aquatics, computers, physical conditioning, community reintegration, spectator events, relaxation exercises, gardening).
- List of adaptive equipment utilized (includes pencil grips, audiobooks, braces, magnifiers, cardholders).
- List of barriers still present at discharge (includes cognitive impairment, paralysis, hearing/vision impairment, spasticity, pain, lack of self-confidence, phobias, motivation, communication impairment, negative attitude, limited ROM).

- Summary of progress achieved during the program.
- Discharge recommendations (includes home programs, social/leisure activities, community resources, adaptive equipment).
- Dates of follow-up or physician's visits.
- Special medical information (includes need for medications, insulin, routine testing).
- Reasons for discharge.

## FORMATIVE AND SUMMATIVE EVALUATIONS

After planning interventions, programs, staff, equipment, materials, facilities, etc., the last step in planning services involves planning evaluation. The TRS must identify, procure, and/or create instruments to collect data; establish a data collection schedule; and determine how and when to adjust client service and program involvement to reflect evaluation findings. **Formative evaluations** during treatment entail immediate decisions about adjusting objectives to accomplish expected results and choosing alternative intervention strategies. **Summative evaluations** after intervention help the TRS evaluate treatment effectiveness for enabling the client to accomplish the results desired. TRSs may re-administer assessment instruments to compare progress achieved to baseline measurements. They may also gather different or new assessment information, use different assessment instruments or processes, and/or redesign the client's individual plan. Short-term (5–30 days) programs include more frequent formative evaluations than longer-term programs. Formative evaluation findings may indicate changing outcome measures or rewriting discharge goals for different program durations following client and team meetings. TRSs may not adjust individual plans when clients are meeting their goals, but just document service and program effectiveness. Client outcome data support efficacy research justifying interventions and evidence-based and ethical practices.

### INTERPRETING FORMATIVE EVALUATIONS

While the TRS is implementing a program for a client, he or she will conduct ongoing **formative evaluations** that will help to identify modifications and adaptations that will improve the experience for the client. Just as ongoing TRS-client interactions inform the treatment process, ongoing TRS-caregiver and/or family interactions also improve caregiver and/or family involvement in the process as it develops. Also, if client progress is not demonstrated, or some unresolved or untreated problems are implied by the emergence of new behaviors, the TRS can obtain helpful input for revising the client's individual plan by networking with other health and human service professionals. Establishing and following activity protocols helps team members organize and document treatment sessions and techniques, promotes consistency, helps clients accomplish goals, and supports communication about program and session progress with colleagues and caregivers. They supply client experience response documentation methods and formative evaluation criteria. By observing client, caregiver, and colleague verbal and nonverbal signals, TRSs collect information on an ongoing basis.

### CONDITIONS FOR SUMMATIVE EVALUATIONS

When a time period specified in a client's plan ends; a program with a specified number of sessions is completed; on a plan-specified date; or when a client/caregiver chooses to terminate the experience, TRSs should make **summative evaluations**, supplementing information they collected about client goals with additional data from client, caregiver, other team member input, and formative evaluations. Research (cf. Austin, 2009) shows consistent/congruent client outcomes are better measured by data from multiple sources. Staff members make referral, discharge, and aftercare recommendations based on these collective data. The purposes of summative evaluation are to determine client progress toward individual plan objectives; measure effectiveness of resource, leadership, and con-tent applications; and assess client satisfaction with the service process and results. Examples of quantitatively and qualitatively comparing initial and subsequent administrations of the same instrument pre- and post-program participation include the Comprehensive Evaluation in Recreation Therapy–Psychiatric/ Behavioral and Physical Disability (CERT–PB, CERT–PD) scales: TRSs record data over time by measurement dates. The Leisure Competence Measure (LCM), using WHO-ICF (World Health Organization International Classification of Functioning) standards and compatible with the FIM (Functional Independence Measure), records progress in multiple areas over time, providing a global database of evidence for intervention efficacy across settings and populations.

## ADJUSTING PROGRAM PARTICIPATION BASED ON DOCUMENTATION

When a TRS's formative evaluations of a client indicate the client will not reach intended outcomes, or the client brings up concerns or displays different behaviors, TRSs may **redefine outcome measures**, rewrite goals, re-administer and/or reanalyze assessments, change or modify program content, change facilitation techniques and/or leadership strategies, change staff assignments or client schedules, add the use of adaptive resources or assistive devices, reconsider colleague and/or caregiver input, redesign the evaluation plan, and change the process of documentation. By revisiting each of the steps taken during planning, the TRS has any or all of these options. If, after revisiting the assessments he or she made of the client initially, the TRS concludes that these correctly identified the client's assets and needs, he or she will then revisit the outcomes of the activity analyses and task analyses and redesign program content and intervention techniques. Conversely, if the TRS finds untreated problems/new client needs after re-interpreting assessment results, he or she accordingly develops a different individualized plan.

## PROGRAM EVALUATION

**Evaluation** is the last phase in planning comprehensive TR/RT service programs, wherein TRSs collect and report data. One purpose of this is to identify which revisions to make in the program. Revising the program makes sure that clients will receive the highest program quality, suitable transitions, and the right kinds of aftercare. Evaluation enables the TRS to obtain information to use for improving program and service delivery and outcomes for clients. The TRS is able to document the benefits realized through application of the TR/RT process. TRSs fulfill their roles as advocates by sharing these benefits with indicated caregivers, supporters, and case managers to facilitate continuity between services and settings. When clients participate in services and programs for longer durations (e.g., months instead of days) and maintaining leisure functioning in inclusive activities is a goal, sharing this information is especially important. TRSs use similar tools and processes to evaluate and improve programs as they do for evaluating IPPs and single therapy session implementation.

### DATA TO COLLECT WHEN EVALUATING COMPREHENSIVE SERVICE PROGRAMS

When evaluating TR/RT service programs, the TRS **collects summative evaluation data** on program content, physical resources, financial resources, management, leadership, and the extent to which the component goals and objectives of the program were met. The TRS and other agency personnel analyze these data and recommend whether to continue the current programs, to modify the existing programs and continue them with those modifications, to discontinue them, or to develop new programs. When the schedule determined ahead of time for a program reaches its natural end, and/or when a client(s) has reached the end of the period of time preplanned for the program, the TRS conducts an evaluation of the service program. The TRS determines the time periods for service programs by referring to accreditation standards, reimbursement protocols, fiscal calendars, and the operation schedules and calendars of other members of the health and human services team, for example hospital clinicians, special educators, and others involved in the delivery of the client's services.

## FOCUSES OF EVALUATION

**Aspects of focus in evaluations** regarding the quality of TR/RT service programs include program efficiency, program effectiveness, and program ethics. Evaluations should answer the questions of whether an analysis of the data gathered on individual clients' plans and on components of the service program indicate that the program content, resources, and leadership benefited the clients and were managed with efficiency and effectiveness. Evaluation answers questions regarding how desirable the clients' program experiences and results were. It also offers evidence to support cause-and-effect relationships between the clients' outcomes and the interventions employed. The TRS uses the information that he or she obtains from the evaluation to inform clinical judgments and decisions. Sources of data that TRSs collect include clients, caregivers, staff members, and administrators. These data include information about resources, staffing, services, and programs. TRSs analyze these data and report them in specialist program reports, program summaries, year-end reports, and annual reports. They present this information and review it with others in staff meetings, professional and lay quality improvement committee sessions, budget preparation meetings, safety audits, and administrative hearings with supervisors.

## REPORTING EVALUATION RESULTS

When TRSs **report evaluation results**, how they present this information can be equally important as what they report. Caregivers anxiously focused on progress may disregard other information. Also, different cultures assign different values to self-determined leisure and independent functioning. Hence TRSs and administrators must tread carefully regarding family caregiving roles, finances, and other sensitive issues. TR/RT evaluation reports are also influenced by factors including financial accountability measures, regulatory agency requirements, quality improvement processes, formal and informal interactions among various health and human services professionals within the particular practice setting, and available computer technology and software support. However, irrespective of all the specific variables that influence the evaluation report, all of these documents that summarize the client's outcomes should contain the following: a brief description of therapeutic goals for the client and measures used for outcomes; a brief overview of program content, modalities, facilitation techniques, and leadership strategies; a list of evaluation tools and assessment instruments; a statement about any concerns or biases in data collection and interpretation; and recommendations for revising, continuing, or discontinuing the program according to client achievement/non-achievement of outcome goals.

# Document Program and Client Incidents

## DOCUMENTING ADVERSE INCIDENTS

Each healthcare facility should have established protocols for **documenting adverse incident,** and the RT must always immediately report any error to a supervisor so that steps can be taken to prevent further problems or injury to the client. An incident report should be filled out to document the adverse incident, initiated by the person involved or closest to the client when the incident occurred. The incident report should include:

- **Name**: The name of the person who is directly involved in or responsible, those affected by the incident, and witnesses.
- **Other identifying information**: Information so that injured parties and witnesses can be identified and contacted, such as birthdates, genders, addresses, and telephone numbers.

- **Time, date, and location**: The exact time, date, and location of the incident. If unknown (such as when a client is found on the floor), the time the incident was discovered and the last time the client was observed should be documented.
- **Narrative**: A description of what happened and any actions taken at the time (such as lifting a client) or as a result of the action (transport to X-ray department).

# Administration

## Maintain Department Documentation

### WRITTEN PLANS OF OPERATION

#### PURPOSE, FUNCTION, CONTENT, AND ELEMENTS

Professional standards of practice require a TR/RT program/agency to have a **written plan of operation** to assure services accomplish intended goals. TRS resource and service management is guided by this plan. It includes information from policy and procedure manuals, governing regulations and codes, executive orders, and recorded meeting minutes. This plan also reflects the mission and goals of the organization. When the only function of an agency is TR/RT, the plan of operation contains all written documents defining services offered and describing procedures for resource and personnel management. While the content of each written plan of operation varies for individual agencies, typical elements of most plans of operation include the agency's vision statement, mission statement, value statement, and goal statement; the organizational structure of the agency; the scope of care offered by the agency; the programs and services the agency offers; the agency protocols; agency procedures; its staff's credentials; its quality improvement measures and processes; its evaluation procedures; and its research procedures and activities.

#### VISION, MISSION, VALUE, PHILOSOPHY, AND GOAL STATEMENTS

A TR/RT agency's **vision statement** defines its beliefs and desired future results. The **mission statement** identifies its unique purpose/raison d'être. While the vision statement describes how the agency will appear if it fulfills its potential, the mission statement clarifies the vision by indicating how the agency's provision of services will change the world. **Goal statements** describe the benefits and results clients will receive from the TR/RT programs or services, supplying direction. The goals connect the vision and mission by stating how the agency will organize its practices to attain its desired future. TR/RT agencies can commit their service to continuous improvement and express their organizational work through writing clear vision, mission, and goal statements. **Value statements** are found with vision and mission statements. They serve as foundations for performance expectations, program direction, organizational change, and client health. They guide TRSs in forming therapeutic relationships and implementing interventions, and managers in operational decision-making. Influenced by regulatory and professional standards, practices, and trends, value statements are reference points describing programs for stakeholders. Some agencies may also have separate **philosophy statements**. These connect services to the vision and mission by identifying fundamental theories, concepts, beliefs, and values regarding outcomes and/or services.

#### ORGANIZATIONAL STRUCTURE, SCOPE OF CARE, AND SERVICES OFFERED

Operation plans obtain **schematic organizational charts** from agency policy and procedure manuals. Structures include special recreation associations whose only function is TR/RT services, TRSs occupying discrete departments within healthcare settings, or TR/RT divisions of public recreation agencies. Charts help TRSs identify formal organizational relationships, responsibility areas, accountable persons, and communication channels. TR/RT service organization must match agency organizational structure. Job descriptions supplement charts, defining specific duties; scope of authority and responsibilities; required qualifications, credentials, and competencies; and reporting relationships. Service unit staffs collectively enable agency mission achievement. Scope of care describes service goals and objectives and establishes complementary organizational structures. Service scope has influences like the Healthy People initiatives, WHO-ICF model, global health care, health information and technology access, accountability demands, cost containment, safety, quality, holistic/integrative health focus, cultural, community, and personal factors. TRS scope of care is shifting from specialized toward multi-skilled and the full care continuum. Scope of care defines programs and services offered. Hospital departments may offer a continuum from inpatient to home services. TRSs develop specific program plans for each service and program identifying the unit goal each supports, plus purpose, goals, interventions, leadership strategies, and outcomes.

## Protocols, Policies, Procedures, and Rules

TR/RT managers create **protocols/intervention plans** for each service area and program. These define best practices for a specific activity with given client needs, standardized based on professional consensus, research literature reviews, or recent research evidence. Agencies typically offer services/programs to clients having similar needs. One protocol type is for a problem area or diagnosis. Another is for a program. Hospitals typically use protocols; outpatient/non-acute care settings usually use intervention plans. While formats can differ, both commonly share referral information, assessment summaries of client strengths and needs, expected outcomes, interventions, and leadership strategies, including risk and safety management measures. TRSs use protocols/intervention plans as blueprints for daily client interactions. Managers use them for documenting TR/RT benefits, assessing staff performance, and developing efficacy studies to standardize practice, create quality improvement plans, and validate best practices. **Policies, procedures, and rules** specify service/program operational directions. In addition to basic P&Ps, program rules may define expected client behaviors and staff-to-client ratios, ensuring consistent, orderly staff performance and daily operations. TR/RT programs need fewer P&Ps/rules within agencies having extensive ones. TR/RT should develop P&Ps/rules minimally required for safe, effective service and client success.

## Guidelines for Equipment Use, Supplies, and Facilities

TRSs working in recreational or healthcare facilities must ensure that therapy and activity participants return sports, kitchen, and other equipment to their storage locations after use, clean up kitchen or picnic activity areas, and ask TRSs or other TR/RT staff to access stored gym equipment. TR/RT staff must make monthly safety checks of all supplies and equipment in TR/RT facilities. They are responsible for monitoring kitchen refrigerator temperatures; enforcing the containment, labeling, and dating of foods in kitchens; and disposing of foods if they are not appropriately contained/labeled/dated. TRSs are in charge of scheduling TR/RT picnic shelter, kitchen, weight room, and gym time with hospital or clinic patient groups, inpatient and outpatient programs, staff groups, and units, with patient groups receiving priority. Patient or staff groups that want to schedule additional activities not included in the facility's master schedule must clear these with the TRS or other TR/RT staff member who is designated in charge of scheduling.

## Quality Improvement

**Quality improvement (QI) programs** constitute one method for evaluating comprehensive TR/RT services and programs. Agency protocols and mission statements typically contain QI indicators, which provide benchmarks or targets for identifying areas needing improvement and for measuring program effectiveness. When a TRS collects data systematically on a specific group(s) of clients for the purpose of documenting program and service effectiveness, the benefits of service delivery are determined through efficacy research. Efficacy research studies examine how program content, physical resources, financial resources, management, and leadership interact with each other and how they are related to outcomes for clients. Case studies of individual clients, quality improvement reviews, quality improvement audits, and monitoring and revision of critical pathways all contribute to the measurement and documentation of program effectiveness. It is of critical importance to report program outcomes and effectiveness because third-party payers and other external reviewers are placing increasing emphasis and attention on whether specific services contribute to the efficiency and effectiveness of intervention.

## CONTINUOUS QUALITY IMPROVEMENT (CQI)

The Joint Commission shifted healthcare quality assurance (QA) to outcome-oriented measures in the 1990s, emphasizing ongoing measurement of processes improving outcomes, which it designated **continuous quality improvement (CQI) and performance improvement (PI).** Client safety gained primary focus in the early 2000s, supported by evidence-based and QI practices. The 2005 Patient Safety and Quality Improvement Act encouraged stakeholder collaboration for improving quality by reducing mistakes and disseminating greater knowledge to all constituents. Total quality management (TQM) is an approach combining cost containment with raising care value. CQI and/or PI are elements of TQM, which also emphasizes client-oriented approaches, client satisfaction, empowering employees, structured problem-solving, and teamwork. TQM acknowledges change is ongoing and embraces change. Systematic measurement of indicators and outcomes, discerning values important to service delivery, is required for continuous improvement of care safety and quality. CQI/PI indicators are measurable care/service components reflecting quality. Structure indicators include policy compliance, correct equipment use, and adequate staffing. Process indicators include professional practice guidelines, client-therapist interactions, and consensus about intervention efficacy. Outcome indicators measure intervention effects on client health relative to environmental and personal variables.

## UTILIZATION REVIEW

A significant consideration for TRSs is that program/agency quality improvement teams may not be familiar/directly experienced with TR/RT standards of practice and efficacy research. TR/RT managers, TRSs and other staff must communicate pertinent research evidence and theories supporting TR/RT intervention practices, results, and benefits. Managers design quality improvement plans, including them in their program/agency operational manuals. One element of a quality improvement program is a set of procedures identifying how client case studies and/or patient charts will be reviewed for documenting necessity and effectiveness of services. A **utilization review** is a process agencies and administrators apply to ensure care is effective and services medically necessary. Concurrent reviews occur during service, retrospective reviews following service. Utilization reviews investigate how often an intervention is scheduled (frequency), how long each intervention lasts (duration), and whether physical rehabilitation is indicated or specialized services (intensity). This information is used to assure services can be reasonably expected to improve client functioning.

## PEER REVIEW AND OUTCOME MONITORING

**Peer review** is an intensive process in which an RT is reviewed by like practitioners. Peer review is often triggered by root cause analysis that indicates the need to focus on an individual or may be part of routine evaluation. A ranking system is usually used to indicate compliance with standards:

- Care is based on standards and typical of that provided by like practitioners.
- Variance may occur in care, but outcomes are satisfactory.
- Care is not consistent with that provided by like practitioners.
- Variance resulted in negative outcomes.

**Outcome monitoring** is the periodic assessment of a program, including inputs and outputs. Outcome monitoring does not require benchmarks or comparison groups and does not determine what intervention resulted in an outcome and cannot predict risk behaviors, but can track changes associated with interventions. Data must be collected in at least 2 different time periods. Outcome monitoring is used to improve the effectiveness of programs by determining what appears to work and what does not.

## Cost-Benefit Analysis

A **cost-benefit analysis** uses average cost of an event and the cost of intervention to demonstrate savings.

- For example, computer repair costs related to improper computer use are $125/hour. If the institution averages 20 hours of computer repair a month ($125 X 20 = $2500) X 12 months ($2500 X 12), the annual cost equals $30,000.
- If the intervention includes staff training materials ($400), instructor costs ($2000) and staff costs ($10,000), the total intervention cost is $400 + $2000 + 10,000 for a total of $12,400.
- If the goal were to decrease repair costs by 80% to 4 hours per month, then savings would be calculated as 4 x $125 = $500 monthly costs X 12 = $6000 subtracted from the current annual cost of $30,000 = $24,000 savings.
- Subtracting the intervention costs from the savings gives the annual cost benefit: $24,000 - $12,400 = $11,600 annual cost benefit.

## Program Evaluation and Accountability

### Attendance and Participation Rates

The process of **program evaluation** and **accountability** are generally formalized with specific forms developed to facilitate evaluation. While formats may vary, common issues to be assessed include:

- Program title and primary function or focus.
- Program purpose and goals and client goals and measurable objectives.
- Client population (multiple or specific client populations).
- Client characteristics for those who would benefit most from the program.
- Decision making process for determining how or if a client might benefit from the program.
- Method of assigning clients.
- Activities utilized in the program in order to meet goals.
- Staff interactions and intervention strategies.
- Program structure (duration, sessions per week, total sessions, individual sessions, number of clients, typical format, and attendance and participation rates (including client compliance and perseverance as well as drop-out rates)
- Program resources (materials, equipment facilities, support services).
- Complaints, incident reports.
- Staffing requirements (numbers, training, education) and client-staff ratio (with comparison to like facilities).

## Fiscal Management

### Payment for TR/RT Services

Practices associated with **paying for TR/RT services** are frequently defined by the federal government. In determining their coverage and payment policies, private health insurance companies then eventually accept and follow these federally established criteria as well. When TR/RT services are delivered in healthcare settings, the federal Centers for Medicare and Medicaid Services (CMS) defines "active treatment" as services a provider delivers according to an individualized assessment and treatment plan, supervised by a medical doctor, and deemed "reasonable and necessary." Private insurers typically reimburse providers for services fitting this federal definition of active treatment. After reviewing claims submitted, they authorize full or partial payment, or deny it. Under capitated employer plans, reimbursement rates are fixed amounts or some expenses are not covered. When insurers underpay, sometimes patients/clients pay the difference; but many doctors, practices, or other practitioners write off the remainder.

## SERVICE PAYMENTS IN PUBLIC AGENCIES

When TRSs provide TR/RT services under the aegis of federal, state, or local government agencies, the revenues for these services are funded by taxes. Funds are allocated annually from federal or state legislatures for federal or state agencies, and from the general funds for city government agencies. To add to these funds, government and nongovernment matching grants may be accessed. The current political and economic climates often bring about changes in the tax bases. As a result, TRSs may unexpectedly sustain decreases or increases in these yearly appropriations. To add to allocations, public agencies charge fee-for-services. These are also charged by for-profit and nonprofit service agencies and camps and other private providers (e.g., The Arc). Fees may cover a part of program costs or their total costs, depending on individual program cost-to-revenue ratio. Some agencies/programs charge yearly membership fees, allowing member access to certain programs at no additional cost and minimal additions for expensive programs such as equestrian or aquatic therapies. Some agencies charge membership fees for clients outside their districts, but not district residents. Agencies may also award scholarships to some participants, and/or base fees on sliding scales according to individual client income/financial status.

## FACTORS INFLUENCING PAYMENT FOR SERVICES

Rising healthcare costs and needs to monitor service delivery have led to managed care options. For instance, health **insurance preferred provider organizations (PPOs)** offer lower prices as incentives for their use, providing services on a fee-for-service basis. The government-mandated **Prospective Payment System (PPS)** establishes pre-arranged reimbursement amounts for specified services from government providers, regardless of actual service cost. Private employers set group insurance coverage and benefit rates. Some employers also capitate employee group payments, limiting them to fixed amounts. In all practice settings, as members of integrated healthcare system teams, TRSs must document TR/RT intervention cost-effectiveness and client outcomes/benefits for insurance companies and clients. This is necessary due to increases in consumer demands, benefit recipients, choices of providers, uninsured client coverage, malpractice insurance costs, technology, complicated reimbursement methods, catastrophic and chronic disease care, and emergency preparedness for natural disasters and bioterrorism, which contribute to a competitive and financially restricted healthcare environment. TRSs have an opportunity to establish a unique niche in the health and human services delivery system relative to current emphases on promoting quality of life behaviors, prevention, and the interrelationship of environmental and personal factors and life activity functioning.

## RATE SETTING FOR TR/RT SERVICES

TR/RT managers may **establish service rates** to charge insurers and clients appropriately. Fees may cover all or part of total expenses. While managed care approaches negotiate amounts including risk-adjustment factors like deductibles, allowances, discounts, etc., other approaches include direct and indirect expenses in total service cost. TRSs can identify direct and indirect service delivery costs through rate-setting, measuring results by what a service actually costs to achieve desired benefits. Accounting for uncollectables and allowances, service prices may be affected by what the market will allow. Salaries, fringe benefits, equipment, supplies, pre-intervention and post-intervention preparation time, paperwork time, etc., are included in direct costs. TRSs and TR/RT departments/units typically share utility costs, maintenance expenses, and other indirect costs required for delivering services with other services using a facility/agency. TRSs establish per-unit cost rates/per-service unit charges. TR/RT services may have hourly rates divided into 15-minute segments. Market trends influence rate variation; hence the American Medical Association (AMA) codes therapies/treatments yearly using Current Procedural Terminology (CPT) codes. Codes do/do not cover TRS interventions depending whether they are found to contribute directly to client care plans. Geographic location/setting influences billing type, TRS salary, and service charge/unit cost.

## BUDGETING

Depending on the setting, TR/RT services can be identified as having an individual budget or as a part of a larger division or department budget. All budgets begin as proposals. Once the designated boards and people approve budget proposals, these become budgets for a year or other defined time period. TRSs have vital roles in the process of preparing budgets and also may serve as advisors to financial departments during budget development, presentation, and approval. Following budget implementation, TRSs are responsible for reconciling quarterly/monthly budget reports and keeping expenditures within approved budget limits. Comptrollers/accountants may consult TRSs during the facility/agency fiscal year. One health and human services budget format is line-item/object-of-expenditure. Every item is assigned its line in the account and frequently a classification number/code, which are similar across settings. The program budget is another format. All income (revenue) and expenses for a whole program are included. Another format is the zero-based budget. Proposed services are ranked by priority for every fiscal year and resources allocated accordingly. TRSs may be requested to use current revenue and expense patterns to estimate the next fiscal year's needs.

### OPERATING BUDGETS

**Operating budget components** are revenues (income) and expenses. Revenues include contracts, charges, fees, insurance reimbursements, and grants. Expenses include employee salaries, equipment, supplies, and overhead. Larger amounts of money for expensive equipment or buildings are capital expenses. Capital expenses are usually separated out into a separate budget, but may also sometimes be incorporated into the main operating budget. Every individual agency or facility establishes what amount constitutes a capital expense. For example, some smaller agencies, facilities, departments, or units may consider capital expenses as anything costing more than $50; larger facilities or agencies may designate capital expenses as anything costing more than $1,000. The time frame for developing an operating budget and the specific procedures to be followed vary according to the individual agency. Some TR/RT agencies first conduct analyses of the revenues and expenses in the previous fiscal year and then assign dollar amounts to every department. Others have their managers request department allocations according to their budget categories.

### BUDGET DEVELOPMENT

At a TR/RT agency, typically the personnel involved in budget planning and development first estimate their necessary expenses for the coming fiscal year and then project the revenues they think they will receive based on their agency budget calendar. During the **process of developing the budget,** the other personnel involved may ask the TRS to reassess the figures he or she has submitted previously for TR/RT services, in order to revise the proposed budget, or to offer more justification for the current budget proposal. Throughout the fiscal year, the TRS may be requested to fill out specified financial forms. For example, committed costs, ongoing costs—employee salaries, rental of the building(s)/space, and insurance coverage—and replacement costs for buying new equipment, all require completing certain forms. TRSs are responsible for knowing impending due dates for submitting these forms and turning them in in a timely way. TRSs are also expected to know which revenues and expenses are related to their delivery of TR/RT services during development of the budget proposal. Hospital/corporation boards of directors, finance committees, or city councils approve proposed budgets depending on the setting.

## APPROVED BUDGET PROPOSALS

Once an agency/facility's governing authority approves a budget proposal, it becomes a legal document as the operating budget. Depending on changes various boards and administrators made before approving it, dollar amounts assigned for each program/category may/may not reflect amounts originally requested. Actual budget allocations are frequently organized to enable generation of monthly reports detailing every budget category's activities. TRS responsibilities may include aligning every account with fiscal year allocations, preventing overspending and assuring the whole budget is balanced by the end of the fiscal year, and/or reconciling specific accounts quarterly/monthly to balance year-end totals. Another TRS responsibility can be keeping specific program records, for example, units and full-time equivalents (FTEs) of time spent in client contact. Forty hours per week or 2080 hours per year equals one FTE. When TRSs regularly conduct financial audits, they can more easily identify accounting errors and project necessary account allocation changes. They also provide managers with cost analysis data for justifying resource allocations and/or documenting program effectiveness.

## FUNDING FOR TR/RT SERVICES

In addition to yearly appropriations from taxpayer revenues, matching grants, and fee-for-services charged to clients, TRSs working in health and human services agencies often depend on other **grants, donations, support** from foundations, gifts, and contracts. Specific options and innovative programs are funded by sources like these. Fundraising and disbursement for specific participants/events may involve TRS collaboration with foundations/advisory committees having tax-exempt 501(c)(3) status. Social service agencies rely on the United Way as a major funding source. Agencies may meet specific financial goals through annual fund drives. For example, TRS managers may submit requests to the United Way, presenting funding needs at budget hearings. United Way personnel evaluate requests according to annual fund drive revenues and funding priorities their board of directors establishes. Successful businesses and wealthy families establish foundations contributing funds. Federal, state, and local governments also offer grants. Managers may have to apply via forms/letters identifying funder benefits for contributing to compete for grants. Community Lion's and Rotary Clubs also sponsor clients and raise funds to buy handicapped-accessible vans for agencies, etc. To finance adventure/challenge therapies, TRSs also may contract for services.

# Assign and Monitor Personnel

## RECRUITING, HIRING, AND ORIENTING NEW TRSS

Managers **advertise TRS openings** using university/college placement services, conference job fairs, newspapers/newsletters, sending opening announcements to agencies providing TRS services, and professional networking. Candidates meeting preset criteria are screened and interviewed on site. Agencies typically require a university/college TR/RT degree or specialization, NCTRC certification, state certification/licensure/registration in states offering these, and the CPRP (Certified Park and Recreation Professional) credential when park and recreation training is needed. Agencies may stipulate specific training and/or coursework in excess of NCTRC requirements. Managers may additionally examine candidates' university/college transcripts for successful completion of certain courses. Managers conduct staff orientations regarding agency expectations, protocols, and specific job duties—either before or during a period of probation.

Orientation includes explaining supervisory processes, performance expectations, review and competency procedures, emergency protocols, personnel policies, preparation of new TRS professional development (PD) plans, initial assessment of required daily task competencies, training needs identification (e.g., technology use), and helping new employees write objectives to serve as the foundations of their PD plans and guidance for their supervisory interactions.

## PERSONNEL SUPERVISION

TR/RT and agency managers perform three kinds of **supervision**: (1) managerial supervision, to ensure comprehension and compliance with agency/department policies and initiatives; (2) clinical supervision, to enhance therapist-client interactions and professional skills; and (3) supportive supervision, to enhance job satisfaction and morale. Any or all of these types of supervision take place during observations, case presentations, performance interviews, quality audits, and journaling. Experts advise that managers should assign clinical supervision to others who ensure and regulate productivity, to keep supervisory boundaries distinct and to keep the focus on the growth and development of the clinical staff. TRSs typically first experience clinical supervision as interns, and continue to receive it throughout their careers to improve the quality of their therapeutic relationships and their intervention skills on a continuing basis. Competency improvement and performance review procedures vary among agencies. However, typically a three- to six-month period of probation is followed by a formal review, with formal reviews repeated annually thereafter. To ensure TRS understanding of employer expectations and prevent surprises during performance reviews, managers should thoroughly discuss performance expectations during recruitment and clearly explain competency assessment plans during orientation periods.

## INTERNSHIPS AND MANAGING INTERNS

Today, students who pursue typical university/college education and training to obtain degrees in TR/RT and prepare for becoming certified TRSs are required to participate in **internship experiences** on a nearly universal basis. The American Therapeutic Recreation Association (ATRA) and other professional TR/RT organizations have published professional guidelines that define their guidelines for managing these internships. The role of the TR/RT or agency manager is to prepare TRSs and other agency staff members to support student interns in learning professional TR/RT practice and making the transition to professional careers as TRSs once they complete their degrees and obtain their certification credentials. Throughout an internship, an intern takes on increasing amounts of responsibility. At the same time, the intern must receive clinical supervision to assist in the process of developing and then letting go of therapeutic relationships. Since entry-level TRSs today are expected to demonstrate effective job performance much sooner upon entering their first professional employment, internships have gained considerable importance and value.

## MANAGING VOLUNTEERS

As healthcare costs have risen, more people have obtained health insurance; providers are obligated to serve others without coverage; practitioner and staff shortages exist; and managed care practices limit expenditures, constraining costs; health and human services and TR/RT agencies/departments realize increased needs and benefits of engaging **volunteers** as a means of adding to their staffing without having to pay additional salaries/wages. Some TRSs acquire volunteers by taking the volunteer management responsibility in their unit/department; others go through the Human Resources department at their facility. Volunteer management activities are similar to those in paid employee management. Volunteers improve services by contributing their time, abilities, skills, and financial and other resources. The natures of the particular clientele and setting influence variations in the roles of volunteers. Some volunteers raise funds, acquire resources, and perform other support duties; some perform or direct service duties. Managers facilitate volunteer recognition programs and develop and monitor volunteer protocols. Manager and staff duties relative to volunteers are influenced by how much their agency utilizes them.

# NCTRC Practice Test

Want to take this practice test in an online interactive format? Check out the online resources page, which includes interactive practice questions and much more: **mometrix.com/resources719/nctrc**

**1. During an initial assessment, the client shows little facial expression or is very slow to show expressions. How would the CTRS document this client's affect?**

   a. Flat
   b. Broad
   c. Blunted
   d. Inappropriate

**2. Which of the following is NOT an essential outcome of rehabilitation therapy for pediatric clients?**

   a. Improved physical health
   b. Reduced complications
   c. Reduced cost of care
   d. Improved skills in coping with hospitalization

**3. According to Havighurst's Theory of Adult Development, which of the following best characterizes middle age?**

   a. Managing a home and finding a congenial social group
   b. Establishing ties with those in the same age group and adjusting to decreased physical strength
   c. Establishing physical living arrangements that are satisfactory
   d. Achieving civil and social responsibility and maintaining an economic standard of living

**4. When choosing a recreational activity for a client, the MOST important consideration is the client's**

   a. interests.
   b. physical abilities.
   c. mental status.
   d. financial resources.

**5. Which of the following video game sports simulation programs is BEST to improve balance and coordination?**

   a. Golfing
   b. Tennis
   c. Hula hoop
   d. Bowling

**6. Which theory states that a change in one family member's behavior will affect others in the family?**

  a. Rosenstock's Health Belief Model
  b. Ajzen's Theory of Planned Behavior
  c. Bowen's Family Systems Theory
  d. Fishbein and Ajzen's Theory of Reasoned Action

**7. Which of the following is NOT acceptable for the continuing education credit required for recertification?**

  a. Completing field-related academic courses
  b. Presenting a lecture at a national recreation therapy conference
  c. Making a poster presentation at a state recreation therapy conference
  d. Taking a CPR course

**8. Which of the following principles in the American Therapeutic Recreation Association (ATRA) Code of Ethics requires that the CTRS use skills to assist clients while respecting the clients' rights to make decisions and preventing harm?**

  a. Beneficence
  b. Nonmaleficence
  c. Autonomy
  d. Justice

**9. Which of the following laws requires that clients in nursing homes be engaged in a program of activities?**

  a. American's with Disabilities Act (ADA)
  b. Older American Act (OAA)
  c. Omnibus Budget Reconciliation Act (OBRA)
  d. Health Insurance Portability and Accountability Act (HIPAA)

**10. Which of the following is NOT an example of adult client advocacy?**

  a. Describing client's apprehensions to other team members
  b. Listening to and observing client to determine needs
  c. Requesting intervention to meet client's needs
  d. Telling family members the client states he is depressed

**11. Beep baseball was primarily designed for those with which type of disability?**

  a. Hearing impairment
  b. Visual impairment
  c. Mental impairment
  d. Paraplegia

**12. Which of the following best describes Kolb's Model of Experiential Learning?**

  a. Knowledge develops from experience interacting with cognition and perception
  b. Knowledge and experience are equally important
  c. Experience precedes knowledge in learning
  d. Learning cannot be acquired without experience and perception

**13. Which is the best solution for a client who has limited mobility and tends to push food from the plate and accidentally shove plates onto the floor?**

a. Assist the client with eating
b. Feed the client
c. Provide a clip-on plate edge and a non-skid plate mat
d. Provide liquids and finger foods only

**14. In Jean Piaget's Theory of Cognitive Development, which stage is characterized by poor logical ability, magical thinking, egocentrism, and beginning to understand cause and effect?**

a. Sensorimotor
b. Preoperational
c. Concrete operational
d. Formal operational

**15. Which of the following is NOT an indication of tactile sensitivity?**

a. Exhibiting distress when hands are dirty
b. Complaining about clothing labels rubbing against the skin
c. Refusing to wear uncomfortable clothing
d. Brushing hair three to four times daily

**16. Pseudohypertrophic (Duchenne) muscular dystrophy is characterized by**

a. muscle weakness, enlarged muscles from fatty infiltration, and joint and other skeletal deformities.
b. weakness in the upper arms, shoulders that are angled forward, and a lack of facial mobility.
c. weakness of proximal muscles of the pelvic and shoulder girdles.
d. weakness of eyelid and throat muscles.

**17. Which of the following is NOT characteristic of placing children with disabilities in the least restrictive environment for study, sports, and recreation?**

a. Placing a child in an environment as close to traditional as possible
b. Discontinuing all self-contained special programs
c. Placing the child according to individual needs
d. Providing alternative choices

**18. Which of the following is an example of normalization for a 20-year-old man with Down Syndrome?**

a. Assisting him in taking a bus independently to attend a movie theater
b. Placing him in a long-term care facility with full-time supervision
c. Refusing to allow him to carry or play with children's toys in public
d. Providing rules for behavior in different situations

**19. A group of adolescents with autistic disorder are going to attend an inclusive summer camp with non-disabled adolescents. Which of the following is the FIRST step?**

a. Provide funding
b. Identify support staff
c. Assess individual needs
d. Provide staff training

**20. A 24-year old woman with cerebral palsy would like to participate in bowling but has poor mobility and cannot maintain balance and swing or throw the bowling ball. Which intervention is MOST appropriate?**

    a. Bowling ball with grip handles
    b. Bradshaw Bowl Buggy
    c. Bowling ball pusher
    d. Bowling ramp

**21. Which of the following is NOT included in the 2004 Individuals with Disabilities Education Act (IDEA)?**

    a. Free appropriate public education
    b. Individualized education programs (IEPs)
    c. Best educational program available
    d. Least restrictive environment

**22. A 70-year-old man with dementia of the Alzheimer type has episodes of extreme agitation and combative behavior two or three times daily. Which of the following is the BEST initial approach?**

    a. Leave the client undisturbed during these periods
    b. Analyze the pattern of agitation
    c. Change support staff
    d. Apply restraints to prevent injury to others

**23. A 45-year-old man with traumatic brain injury exhibits pronounced changes in personality, impulsive risk-taking behavior, and little facial emotion. Which of the following is the most likely site of injury?**

    a. Frontal lobe
    b. Parietal lobe
    c. Occipital lobe
    d. Cerebellum

**24. Which of the following is NOT a characteristic of attention-deficit/hyperactivity disorder (ADHD)?**

    a. Restlessness/agitation
    b. Becoming easily bored
    c. Frequent daydreams
    d. Speech disorder

**25. During a recreational program in a correctional facility, an inmate asks the CTRS if he is married. Which of the following is the best response?**

    a. "Don't ask personal questions."
    b. "Yes, I'm married."
    c. "I'm sorry. I can't discuss personal information."
    d. "Why do you want to know?"

**26. Which of the following is the MOST appropriate initial aid/assistance in teaching a deaf 32-month-old girl how to do an activity?**

    a.  Video
    b.  Doll demonstration
    c.  Sign-language interpreter
    d.  Pictures

**27. Which of the following should be the FIRST step in conflict resolution?**

    a.  Utilize humor and empathy to defuse escalating tensions
    b.  Summarize the issues, outlining key arguments
    c.  Force a resolution
    d.  Allow both sides to present their side of the conflict without bias

**28. Following a traumatic brain injury, a 57-year-old woman has a Functional Independence Measure (FIM) score of 40 on acute hospital admission and 63 on discharge to a rehabilitation facility, with discharge scores in all areas ranging from 3 to 4. What level of independence or care in the facility is MOST indicated by these scores?**

    a.  Complete independence in care
    b.  Modified independence, including use of assistive devices and activity modification
    c.  Supervision only (stand by without physical assistance)
    d.  Minimal to moderate contact assistance (physical assistance)

**29. According to Knowles' Principles of Adult Learning, adult learners tend to be**

    a.  unmotivated.
    b.  lacking in self-direction.
    c.  practical and goal-oriented.
    d.  insecure.

**30. Which members of the recreational therapy teams are responsible for identifying quality performance improvement projects?**

    a.  Administrative staff
    b.  All staff
    c.  Team leaders
    d.  Supervising physicians

**31. Which of the following is the primary purpose of intern supervision?**

    a.  Promoting professional growth/skills and ensuring program integrity
    b.  Providing mentoring
    c.  Establishing a basis for grades
    d.  Identifying errors or incorrect practices

**32. In which part of the APIE process is the treatment plan documented?**

    a.  Assessment
    b.  Plan
    c.  Implementation
    d.  Evaluation

**33. When dealing with clients in a mental health facility, which of the following activities is BEST to evaluate a client's ability to stay on task and concentrate?**

    a. Arts and crafts project
    b. Personal reading
    c. Treadmill walking
    d. Group sing-along

**34. Which of the following statements should be used to document in the subjective portion of SOAP notes that a client refused to participate in an activity?**

    a. "I can't exercise. My foot hurts."
    b. Client limping and avoiding pressure on left foot so is unable to participate in dancing activity. Blister noted on left heel.
    c. Poorly fitted shoes causing friction rub and blisters.
    d. Treat and protect blisters. Obtain properly fitted shoes.

**35. Which of the following comprises the three components of Carol Peterson's Leisure Ability Model of therapeutic recreation?**

    a. Therapy, leisure activities, and counseling
    b. Therapy, counseling, and supervision
    c. Function, treatment, and leisure participation
    d. Treatment, leisure education, and recreation participation

**36. Using a utilitarian ethical standard of "the most good for the most people," which of the following activities should be selected for an afternoon program for 40 clients in a long-term care facility?**

    a. Sing-along
    b. Monopoly game
    c. Video game simulated sports competition
    d. Outdoor walk

**37. Which of the following statements does NOT justify a violation of confidentiality?**

    a. "I hate my father. I wish he were dead."
    b. "I sometimes feel like cutting myself."
    c. "I'm going to kill the man who injured me when I get out of here."
    d. "I'm saving pills at home, so I can take an overdose."

**38. When completing a pre-transfer assessment, which are the three primary factors to consider?**

    a. Weight, extension, and balance
    b. Safety awareness, strength, and cognition
    c. Strength and motivation
    d. Physical, cognitive, and emotional status

**39. A client needs a single-person transfer from a wheelchair into a car, but the wheelchair is not on level ground. Which of the following is the best solution?**

    a. Use two people for the transfer
    b. Brake the wheelchair and block the front wheels
    c. Move the car and wheelchair to a level area
    d. Level the wheels of the wheelchair

**40. When assisting a client with an activity to improve balance, which of the following types of feedback should be provided?**

    a.  Positive, contingent, and motivational
    b.  Positive, negative, and informational
    c.  Positive and motivational
    d.  Contingent, motivational, and informational

**41. Which of the following is the best response for an 18-year-old man with paraplegia who slips onto the floor but is able to pull himself onto the bed without help and with no injury?**

    a.  "You were very brave."
    b.  "You used good problem-solving skills."
    c.  "You should have called for help."
    d.  "I'm so sorry you had to go through that!"

**42. A client repeatedly uses passive-aggressive behavior such as arriving late for activities, making demands, complaining, and over-sleeping. These behaviors are interfering with progress. Which of the following referrals is most appropriate?**

    a.  Counseling
    b.  Assertiveness training
    c.  Anger management
    d.  Stress management

**43. In Erikson's Psychosocial Development Model, which of the following stages is characteristic of those 6 to 12 years old?**

    a.  Trust vs mistrust
    b.  Autonomy vs shame/doubt
    c.  Industry vs inferiority
    d.  Intimacy vs isolation

**44. Which of the following is an early sign of mild to moderate lithium toxicity?**

    a.  Shakiness, diarrhea, and vomiting
    b.  Agitation and decreased urination
    c.  Agitation and double vision
    d.  Seizures and loss of consciousness

**45. When a client with paraplegia is doing a wheelchair pressure release by leaning side to side, how long should the client take the weight off one side before returning to neutral position?**

    a.  20 to 30 seconds
    b.  25 to 40 seconds
    c.  25 to 60 seconds
    d.  30 to 90 seconds

**46. The CTRS is planning an exercise program for a client with Raynaud's syndrome. Which of the following is correct?**

    a.  She should exercise in a warm environment
    b.  She should limit exercise to less than 30 minutes
    c.  She should do only passive exercises
    d.  She should avoid exercises that involve use of the arms

**47. A client with a T6 spinal cord injury has been sitting in his wheelchair for three hours after lunch and suddenly develops sweating, flushing above the level of injury, a severe headache, nasal congestion, anxiety, and nausea. Which of the following is the most likely cause?**

    a. Flu
    b. Autonomic dysreflexia
    c. Food poisoning
    d. Urinary infection

**48. Which of the following is the correct method to screen a four-year-old child for hearing loss?**

    a. Auditory brainstem response (ABR)
    b. Visual reinforcement audiometry (VRA)
    c. Conditioned play audiometry (CPA)
    d. Standard audiometry

**49. Field observation would be included in which of the following components of Van Andel, Carter, and Robb's Therapeutic Recreation Service Delivery Model?**

    a. Diagnosis/needs and assessments
    b. Treatment/rehabilitation
    c. Education
    d. Prevention/health promotion

**50. What is a good strategy for helping an elderly client overcome feelings of low self-esteem related to chronic illness and loss of autonomy?**

    a. Praise the client constantly for any activities.
    b. Tell the client she has no reason to feel so depressed.
    c. Provide opportunities for the client to make decisions.
    d. Avoid talking to the client about her feelings.

**51. Which of the following is the best method to evaluate a client's educational outcomes after teaching a procedure?**

    a. Ask the client to do a demonstration
    b. Ask the client for feedback
    c. Give the client an oral test
    d. Give the client a written test

**52. The timed-up-and-go (TUG) test is used to assess**

    a. muscle strength.
    b. cognitive status.
    c. mobility and risk of falls.
    d. walking speed.

**53. When converting to computerized record keeping, the MOST important consideration when deciding where to place computer terminals is that the terminals should be**

    a. easily accessed.
    b. placed at point of care.
    c. positioned so the CTRS can enter information while standing.
    d. placed where others cannot read notes being written.

**54. Which of the following disorders is characterized by personality disintegration and distortion in the perception of reality, thought processes, and social development?**

    a. Major depressive disorder
    b. Bipolar disorder
    c. Schizophrenia
    d. Narcissistic personality disorder

**55. Which of the following is NOT typical of addictive behavior?**

    a. Obsession with acquiring the addictive substance
    b. Denial of addiction
    c. Compulsive use of addictive substance
    d. Speaking about addiction

**56. Which of the following play therapy theories or methods focuses on treating specific symptoms or behavioral problems?**

    a. Prescriptive play therapy
    b. Filial therapy
    c. Theraplay
    d. Cognitive behavioral play therapy

**57. Which of the following leisure theories states that people tend to engage in leisure activities that are different from their work experience?**

    a. Spillover theory
    b. Compensation theory
    c. Relaxation theory
    d. Generalization theory

**58. A 17-year-old girl with a history of anorexia and depression is taking topiramate to control generalized tonic-clonic seizures. Which side effect associated with topiramate is of MOST concern?**

    a. Initial sedation
    b. Anorexia and weight loss
    c. Increased appetite and weight gain
    d. Dulling of cognition

**59. What is the FIRST step in an activity task analysis?**

    a. Determine desired outcomes
    b. Divide the activity into component parts
    c. Determine the tasks the client needs to do
    d. Devise methods to assist the client in completing each component

**60. Which of the following programs provides discounted rates for those on Medicare who choose health care providers from a list of those who have agreed to accept Medicare assignment?**

    a. Medicare Managed Care
    b. Prospective Payment System (PPS)
    c. Private insurance pay-for-service
    d. Preferred Provider Organization (PPO)

61. A Hispanic nurse working at an urban hospital was involved in an automobile accident and lost her job and health insurance. Which of the following barriers to care is most likely to prevent her from obtaining therapy?

a. Organizational
b. Geographic
c. Linguistic
d. Socioeconomic

62. Which of the following is NOT an element of an accessible environment?

a. High check-in counters
b. Chairs with adjustable seat and arm heights
c. Light and sound alarm systems
d. Sensitivity training

63. A client who is visually impaired needs to go to another room in the facility and asks for assistance to get there. Which of the following is the correct procedure to assist the client?

a. Hold the client's arm
b. Offer an arm to the client
c. Suggest transportation by wheelchair
d. Walk beside the client and give directions

64. Which of the following is NOT an appropriate source of assessment data?

a. Husband's report of client's condition
b. Telephone interview of friend and neighbor
c. Copy of hospital records
d. Staff report

65. A client with diabetes has been limping and examination shows a small open sore on her great toe. Which of the following initial actions is MOST important?

a. Advise the client to see a physician.
b. Apply a loose protective dressing.
c. Advise the client to get properly fitted shoes.
d. Advise the client to wear a soft slipper on that foot.

66. When working to increase exercise tolerance in a client with chronic obstructive pulmonary disease (COPD), one of the primary goals is an inspiration/expiration ratio of

a. 1:1.
b. 2:1.
c. 1:2.
d. 1:4.

67. When working with a client who is HIV positive, which of the following precautions is necessary?

a. Wear a gown and gloves at all times
b. Wear gloves for contact with bodily fluids
c. Wear gloves, gown, and mask at all times
d. Wear gloves, gown, and mask for all contact with bodily fluids

**68. Which of the following health and human services models focuses on groups, rather than individuals, and their opportunities for achieving good health and a sense a wellbeing as a basic right of human beings?**

   a.  Medical Model
   b.  Community Model
   c.  Psychosocial Rehabilitation Model
   d.  Public Health Model

**69. In considering social psychological aspects of recreation, carrying capacity refers to**

   a.  the maximum weight clients can carry.
   b.  the amount of use an organism can withstand before deterioration.
   c.  the number of people in a given space.
   d.  the maximum number of people or interactions tolerated.

**70. According to Tuckman's model for group interaction, which of the following stages refers to the period during which people develop a sense of trust and are able to communicate ideas and make progress?**

   a.  Forming
   b.  Storming
   c.  Norming
   d.  Performing

**71. When assigning pairs for a get-acquainted activity with a new group of clients, the CTRS states that Jaime, a Hispanic man, and Ming, a Chinese woman, shouldn't be paired together because their cultures are too different and they will be uncomfortable. This is an example of**

   a.  prejudice.
   b.  stereotyping.
   c.  bias.
   d.  discrimination.

**72. When developing an arts-based therapeutic recreation program that meets three times a week for two hours for a group home with 12 adult clients with mild to moderately severe cognitive impairment, which is the best approach?**

   a.  Provide group activities with individual accommodations
   b.  Provide group activities in which all can participate
   c.  Provide different group activities to correspond to cognitive abilities
   d.  Focus on arts and crafts rather than fine arts

**73. Which of the following is an example of a therapeutic recreation leisure service?**

   a.  Adapted swimming lessons for children with disabilities
   b.  A class to help autistic adolescents learn better social skills
   c.  Microwave cooking for those with limited mobility
   d.  Balance exercises for stroke patients

**74. In an interdisciplinary program, helping people manage activities of daily living, such as dressing, bathing, and preparing food is the primary focus of which of the following professionals?**

a. Rehabilitation therapist
b. Occupational therapist
c. Physical therapist
d. Psychologist

**75. Which of the following types of budgets is used for remodeling, repairing, and purchasing equipment or buildings?**

a. Operating budget
b. Capital budget
c. Cash balance budget
d. Master budget

**76. A manager who follows organizational rules exactly and expects everyone else to do so is what type of leader?**

a. Bureaucratic
b. Autocratic
c. Democratic
d. Charismatic

**77. Which of the following is the primary goal of risk management?**

a. Identify potential risks and provide plans to reduce risks
b. Manage problems that arise
c. Provide staff education to reduce risk
d. Document accountability regarding risk factors

**78. Which assessment tool for dementia involves remembering and repeating the names of three common objects and drawing the face of a clock with all 12 numbers and hands indicating the time specified by the examiner?**

a. Mini-Mental State Examination (MMSE)
b. Mini-Cog
c. Digit Repetition Test
d. Confusion Assessment Method

**79. Which of the following is the MOST accurate statement regarding David Austin's Health Improvement/Health Promotion (HI/HP) model?**

a. The stability tendency and the actualization tendency both operate equally throughout therapy
b. The stability tendency lessens as a client gains optimal health and moves toward actualization
c. The stability tendency increases as the client gains freedom of choice and optimal health
d. The actualization tendency decreases and stability tendency increases as the client moves toward optimal health

**80. After initial assessment of a client, the CTRS develops a treatment plan that includes the goal of improving physical condition. Which of the following is the best measurable objective to support this goal?**

a. Exercising regularly
b. Lifting weights daily
c. Signing up for an aerobic dance class
d. Walking for 30 minutes, five times a week

**81. The National Inclusion Project sponsors "Let's All Play" summer camps that include both disabled and non-disabled children, with some accommodations provided so that all can participate. This is an example of which of the following?**

a. Adaptive recreation
b. Holistic recreation
c. Recreative experience
d. Inclusive recreation

**82. The CTRS is assigned to work individually with a new client, whom she recognizes as a fellow member of Alcoholics Anonymous. Which issue does this present?**

a. Conflict of interest
b. Boundary violation
c. Dual relationship
d. Confidentiality

**83. When evaluating the reliability of an assessment tool, which of the following is MOST important?**

a. Ability to measure as intended
b. Scoring consistency with different CTRSs
c. Absence of bias in assessments
d. Staff preference

**84. The ASIA impairment scale is used to assess**

a. cognitive impairment.
b. emotional disorders.
c. spinal cord injury.
d. brain injury.

**85. The CTRS is using the Play Interaction Checklist to assess the social interaction of a five-year-old child. Which of the following is NOT an element of this assessment?**

a. Observing the child with a group of familiar peers
b. Conducting a series of observations
c. Observing other three-year-old children for comparison
d. Engaging the children in conversation

**86. Which of the following assessment tools is MOST appropriate for a 70-year-old client recovering from a stroke to determine her skills (including motor, communication, sensory, cognitive, locomotion, and behavior) prior to developing an activity plan?**

    a. Leisure Diagnostic Battery (LDB)
    b. Leisure Motivation Scale (LMS)
    c. Comprehensive Evaluation in Recreational Therapy (CERT)—Physical Disabilities
    d. Leisure Satisfaction Measure (LSM)

**87. Which of the following is NOT included in the CTRS's scope of practice, according to the NCTRC?**

    a. Assessment
    b. Implementation
    c. Evaluation
    d. Prescription

**88. The purpose of a functional vision assessment for a child is to determine the**

    a. ability to use vision in functioning.
    b. degree of vision impairment.
    c. cause of vision impairment.
    d. ability to function without vision.

**89. Which of the following behavioral observations CANNOT be an indication of depression or withdrawal?**

    a. Broad affect
    b. Slumping posture
    c. Failure to make eye contact
    d. Turning away from interviewer

**90. Which of the following was the primary motivation for founding ATRA and splitting from NTRS in 1984?**

    a. Desire to increase interaction and participation with the health care industry
    b. Lack of a national organization for recreation therapists
    c. Desire to improve financial situation
    d. Desire to focus on recreation as a basic human need

**91. According to the literature on lifespan human growth and development, during what periods do people most demonstrate a desire for more autonomy?**

    a. Adolescence and young adulthood
    b. Infancy and early elementary years
    c. Middle adult and old-age adulthood
    d. The toddler years and adolescence

**92. In the "nature/nurture" debate, nature represents _____ and nurture represents _____.**

    a. heredity; environment
    b. environment; heredity
    c. personalities; behavior
    d. neglecting; educations

**93. Which of the following is most accurate about the role of infant crying in development?**

    a. Crying is a reflex with no other known purpose

    b. Crying's only purpose is to meet physical needs

    c. Crying aids development regardless of response

    d. Crying prompts responses required for survival

**94. Freud's psychoanalytic theory of personality focuses on which aspect of development?**

    a. Archetypal

    b. Psychogenic

    c. Psychosocial

    d. Psychosexual

**95. Who is best known for the theory that humans learn by observing the behaviors of others and the consequences of those behaviors, and then remembering and imitating those behaviors?**

    a. Albert Bandura

    b. B. F. Skinner

    c. Lawrence Kohlberg

    d. Lev Vygotsky

**96. Which choice best orders these personality trait theorists in order of the theorist identifying the fewest traits to the theorist identifying the most traits?**

    a. Allport; Cattell; McCrae & Costa; Eysenck

    b. Eysenck; McCrae & Costa; Cattell; Allport

    c. Cattell; Eysenck; Allport; McCrae & Costa

    d. McCrae & Costa; Cattell; Allport; Eysenck

**97. Which of the following is most accurate about TR according to the medical model?**

    a. Treatment is holistic for broadest client needs

    b. TR is independent of diagnosis or prescription

    c. The role of the RT is determined by the doctor

    d. This model is used most in community settings

**98. In terms of their approach to clients, which health and human services models are the most opposite?**

    a. The recovery model vs. the person-centered model

    b. The custodial model vs. the long-term care model

    c. The health promotion model vs. the wellness model

    d. The medical model vs. the person-centered model

**99. What best defines the relationship between the ICD-10 and the ICF?**

    a. They are entirely unrelated classifications

    b. They are nearly synonymous alternatives

    c. They are complementary to one another

    d. They are mutually exclusive alternatives

**100. Which population category increased the most from 2010 to 2020 according to US census data?**

a. Black/African American
b. Multiple races
c. Hispanic/Latino
d. White non-Hispanic

**101. Experts find that TR expertise must include multicultural competencies to provide relevant and enlightened services. Of four competency divisions, under which area is RTs' knowing how their own cultural values and biases influence interactions with diverse clients?**

a. Knowledge
b. Awareness
c. Skills
d. Relationship

**102. When applying systems theory to doing therapy with groups, which group systems concept is most reflected by the power structure of decision-making (aside from therapist direction) in a given group?**

a. What coalitions have formed in the group
b. What roles different group members play
c. Whether group boundaries admit new data
d. How members of the group communicate

**103. Which of the following is true about dementia symptoms?**

a. Parkinson's disease does not cause dementia, while Alzheimer's disease does
b. Organ failure, as with the kidneys or liver, is not associated with dementia
c. Traumatic brain injury can cause intellectual disabilities but not dementias
d. Parkinson's disease, Alzheimer's disease, organ failure, and TBI can lead to the symptoms of dementias

**104. For which of the following conditions would TR most encourage the use of gross motor skills?**

a. Cerebral Palsy
b. Spinal cord injury
c. Multiple Sclerosis
d. Muscular Dystrophy

**105. What is most accurate about TR with a patient who has had suffered from heart attack(s)?**

a. The role of TR includes physical activity without limits
b. The role of TR includes only limited physical activities
c. The role of TR includes activities for a healthy lifestyle
d. The role of TR includes activities that are not physical

## 106. Which of the following is classified as an endocrine disorder?
  a. Phenylketonuria (PKU)
  b. Polycystic ovary syndrome
  c. Hemochromatosis
  d. Cystic Fibrosis

## 107. Insects can be vectors of infectious diseases. Which type of disease(s) do insects carry and transmit to human hosts?
  a. Diseases from parasites
  b. Diseases from bacteria
  c. Diseases from all these
  d. Diseases from viruses

## 108. If a person's audiological examination shows a hearing loss of 41-55 dB in the better ear (without a hearing aid), this degree of hearing loss is categorized as
  a. mild.
  b. severe.
  c. moderate.
  d. profound.

## 109. If someone is considered legally blind, what does this mean?
  a. The person may be able to see light, shapes, colors, and objects
  b. The person may be able to distinguish lightness from darkness
  c. The person may be able to see light and shapes, but not colors
  d. The person may as well be blind, as he or she cannot see anything

## 110. Which of the following mental health disorders can cause hallucinations and delusions?
  a. Schizophrenia
  b. Bipolar disorder
  c. Major depression
  d. All these can do so

## 111. Which of the following is true about substance abuse and other addictions?
  a. Anyone using sufficient discipline can prevent and/or quit an addiction
  b. Addiction is an illness, and as such it can be treated and even reversed
  c. Before an addict can begin to recover, he or she must first "hit rock bottom"
  d. In order for treatment to work, an addict must be motivated to recover

## 112. Which of the following is the most accurate definition of normalization for people with disabilities?
  a. Getting people with disabilities to appear as normal as it is possible
  b. Giving disabled people equal opportunities based on cultural norms
  c. Making people with disabilities engage in behaviors that are normal
  d. Encouraging people with disabilities to interact with their age peers

**113. The Architectural Barriers Act (ABA) of 1968 requires federally funded facilities to assure access by all people to their buildings. One federal agency responsible for standards to enforce this law is the Department of Housing and Urban Development (HUD). Which of the following agencies is NOT also responsible for these standards?**

a. The Department of Health and Human Services (HHS)
b. The General Services Administration (GSA)
c. The United States Postal Service (USPS)
d. The Department of Defense (DOD)

**114. In the history of the United Nations' efforts to change societal attitudes toward disability, which was the most recent?**

a. The Declaration on the Rights of Disabled Persons (GA, UN)
b. The UN Convention on the Rights of Persons with Disabilities
c. The General Assembly's adoption of the UN's Standard Rules
d. The World Programme of Action concerning Disabled Persons

**115. Which of the following pieces of legislation was first passed the earliest (i.e., not counting amendments, reauthorizations, or updates)?**

a. The IDEA and ADA were passed the same year
b. The Americans with Disabilities Act (the ADA)
c. The IDEA, originally passed as Public Law 94-142
d. The legislation of the Older Americans Act (OAA)

**116. The NCTRC has been recognized by**

a. the Joint Commission.
b. the CMS (Centers for Medicare and Medicaid Services).
c. the CARF (Commission for Accreditation of Rehabilitation Facilities).
d. all of these centers and commissions.

**117. Which of the following proposes that leisure play and recreation help us build up energy for use during our working time?**

a. The Surplus Energy Theory of Herbert Spencer
b. Moritz Lazarus' Recreation/Re-creation theory
c. Recapitulation in Stanley Hall's theory of play
d. Instinctual practice in Karl Groos' play theory

**118. When considering social and psychological aspects of leisure, a definition of leisure as a state of mind (rather than as time or activity) depends on at least four factors. Which of these factors is most closely related to the concept of self-efficacy?**

a. Intrinsic motivation
b. Perceived competence
c. Perceived freedom
d. Positive affect

**119. When considering recreation across the lifespan and the world, research has found which of the following in comparing the recreation of children in American and Thailand?**

a. American children spent more time on TV and internet, Thai children on radio and reading
b. American children spent more time on all recreational categories than Thai children spent
c. Thai children spent more time with TV, radio, internet, and reading than American children
d. Thai children spent less time watching TV than American children and more time in reading

**120. Research comparing active and passive leisure lifestyles has shown which of the following regarding the lifetime social economic costs of being sedentary?**

a. They are greater than those of smoking
b. They are greater than those of heavy drinking
c. They are equal to those of smoking or drinking
d. They are less than those of smoking or drinking

**121. In the SOAP charting method, where would the physician's diagnosis of the patient's problem be?**

a. In the "A" part
b. In the "S" part
c. In the "P" part
d. In the "O" part

**122. "Pt. is 72 yr. old male, 6'1", 172 lbs." This note would be charted where according to the SOAP method?**

a. O of SOAP
b. P of SOAP
c. A of SOAP
d. S of SOAP

**123. What was the purpose for developing the Functional Independence Measure (FIM)?**

a. To increase the options for types of disability and rehabilitation measurement
b. To make measurements and data of disability and rehabilitation more uniform
c. To generate larger amounts of disability and rehabilitation measurement data
d. To make the measurement of disability and rehabilitation data more versatile

**124. Which of the following is true about the Functional Independence Measure (FIM)?**

a. It must be completed through a conference
b. It must be completed through observation
c. It can be completed via telephone interviews
d. It can be completed in any of these manners

**125. What dimensions have been identified in the Functional Independence Measure (FIM)?**

a. Motor
b. Cognitive
c. (A) and (B)
d. Psychosocial

**126. When RTs (or anyone) write measurable objectives for a patient care plan, they should identify who the patient is. What else should they include and not include?**

a. What instruments will measure progress but not patient awareness
b. When results are expected but criteria for results are not necessary
c. What results are desired rather than how they should be measured
d. What criteria are identified for success but not when it should occur

**127. According to the US Census for 2020, what impact did COVID have on the average time spend on leisure and sporting activities when compared to 2019?**

a. Leisure time increased in 2020 due to COVID lock downs
b. Leisure time decreased in 2020 due to COVID restrictions
c. Leisure time remained the same from 2019 to 2020
d. The most common leisure activity in 2020 was playing games and computer use.

**128. In recent years, the most emphasis in selecting specific TR activities for clients has been on**

a. providing activities to the client
b. providing enjoyment to a client
c. producing outcomes for clients
d. all these are equally important

**129. Which of these is NOT one of three important concepts associated with activity analysis and selecting TR activities for clients?**

a. Causality
b. Replicability
c. Intelligibility
d. Predictability

**130. People with spinal cord injuries can participate in rafting and they can enjoy kayaking or canoeing with only minimal adaptations. Which of the following is true about other water sports for people with spinal disabilities?**

a. People with disabilities can water-ski with modifications
b. No known modifications exist for scuba diving by the disabled
c. No known modifications exist for sailing by the disabled
d. Disabled people require no adaptations to enjoy rowing

**131. For a client who knows how to perform many different leisure activities and cooperates and interacts well with others, but is timid about initiating group activities and wants to improve leadership behaviors, which type of RT intervention would be most appropriate?**

a. Leisure skill development
b. Training for social skills
c. Assertiveness training
d. Stress management

**132. When patients have sustained disabling injuries, which of these is true about the leisure education their RT can give them?**

    a. Those with good prior problem-solving skills need no new ones
    b. Learning to advocate for oneself is included in leisure education
    c. RTs can teach disability rights, but not coping with discrimination
    d. RTs teach time and energy management rather than adjustment

**133. Regarding the nature and diversity of recreation and leisure activities, what is NOT accurate?**

    a. It is not acceptable to exclude people based on their race or ethnicity
    b. It is never acceptable to exclude anyone by gender/sexual orientation
    c. Exclusion of certain groups on the basis of medical history is necessary
    d. Individuals or groups must not be excluded due to employment status

**134. In TR program design, Content and Process Descriptions (CPDs) clarify which specific behaviors will serve as evidence that the client has achieved _____ of the program.**

    a. the Terminal Program Objective (TPO)
    b. the Performance Measures (PMs)
    c. the Enabling Objectives (EOs)
    d. all of these components

**135. Of the following types of service delivery systems wherein TR services are delivered, which two are most often combined in government agencies?**

    a. Leisure Services and Health Services
    b. Health Services and Human Services
    c. Human Services and Education Services
    d. Education Services and Leisure Services

**136. Among members of an interdisciplinary team, certain professions are more likely to collaborate with RTs on the levels of program development, implementation, service delivery, and daily planning. Which profession is more likely to work with RTs on the level of the team, but not the other levels named here?**

    a. Occupational therapists
    b. Physical therapists
    c. Music therapists
    d. Art therapists

**137. Which of the following is true about the Prospective Payment System (PPS) in health care service delivery, including TR service delivery?**

    a. Prices are established after the services have been delivered
    b. Prices established may not include all of the services provided
    c. Prices set are not changed by actual costs for the current year
    d. Some additional settlements or payments may be determined

**138. RTs, like other health care professionals, must make accurate documentation of services. One reason for this is to satisfy demands for the professionals' accountability. Which of the following correctly represents another reason?**

    a. Accurate documentation supplies data for efficacy research and quality improvement
    b. Accurate documentation is unrelated to ensuring the quality of the services delivered
    c. Accurate documentation will not help various staff members to communicate better
    d. Accurate documentation is important but not required in terms of the administration

**139. Of the following, which is correct about evaluating a TR/RT program?**

    a. Program evaluation has little impact on service and management decisions
    b. Program evaluation can prove accountability for the donors to the program
    c. Program evaluation is separate from assessing TR/RT program effectiveness
    d. Program evaluation is unlikely to inform the design of future TR/RT programs

**140. Risk management is one quality improvement technique. Among risk management objectives, which of these are pre-loss objectives rather than post-loss objectives?**

    a. Decreasing anxieties and meeting agency legal obligations
    b. Ensuring agency survival and continuing agency operation
    c. Stabilizing agency earnings and continuing agency growth
    d. Minimizing the impact of loss on other people and society

**141. In developing a TR program, which of these sequences the named components correctly?**

    a. Conceptualization, Analysis, Comprehensive Program Goals, Mission Statement
    b. Mission Statement, Comprehensive Program Goals, Analysis, Conceptualization
    c. Comprehensive Program Goals, Conceptualization, Mission Statement, Analysis
    d. Analysis, Conceptualization, Mission Statement, Comprehensive Program Goals

**142. Which of the following is accurate regarding NCTRC requirements for internship?**

    a. Internship must be at least 10 hours a week but not over 25 hours a week
    b. Internship must be at least 20 hours a week but not over 45 hours a week
    c. Internship can be completed at more than one agency or several agencies
    d. Internship requires a minimum of 10 consecutive weeks and/or 400 hours

**143. What is a result of managed care payments for TR services?**

    a. Managed care has not affected determining and justifying service needs
    b. Providers of TR/RT services no longer have to prove patient service needs
    c. Authority for determining patient service needs was shifted to providers
    d. Authority for determining patient service needs has moved to the payer

**144. Which of these is accurate regarding management of TR facilities and equipment?**

    a. Accessibility standards are the same for all TR areas
    b. Accessibility standards dictate specific ramp grades
    c. Accessibility standards exclude any mention of signs
    d. Accessibility standards are not applicable to parking

**145. Historically, TR emerged through which of these influences most?**

    a.  Medical and health care reform movements more than social reform movements

    b.  Military hospitals in world wars rather than public and private hospitals and clinics

    c.  The development of the Playground Movement that took place from 1850 to 1920

    d.  All these were factors that contributed in equal amounts to the emergence of TR.

**146. To receive certification as a Certified Therapeutic Recreation Specialist (CTRS), which of these is an academic requirement?**

    a.  18 semester hours in TR and Recreation plus 18 semester hours supportive course work

    b.  18 semester hours, 12 in TR and the rest in Recreation at an accredited college/university

    c.  Courses in anatomy and physiology and human services, but not in abnormal psychology

    d.  A major in TR only; majoring in Recreation with an option in TR is not permitted for CTRS

**147. Which statement is accurate regarding how RTs in clinical settings advocate for disabled clients?**

    a.  RT patient advocacy in clinical settings does not include transportation resources

    b.  If a patient's knowledge of recreational opportunities is limited, RTs address this

    c.  Access to facilities for patients with disabilities is advocated by other professions

    d.  RTs advocate physical facility access, but not attitudinal obstacles to the disabled

**148. Regarding the ATRA Code of Ethics, which of these is defined under the principle of competence?**

    a.  The TR professional's expanding his or her practice knowledge

    b.  The TR professional's responsibilities for doing both (A) and (C)

    c.  The TR professional's contribution to advancing the profession

    d.  The TR professional's competence is not in this Code of Ethics

**149. A RT who wants to provide TRS to individuals on the autism spectrum disorder can obtain a specialty certification in which of these?**

    a.  Developmental Disabilities

    b.  Behavioral Health Services

    c.  Community Inclusion Services

    d.  Physical Medicine/Rehabilitation

**150. When a college or university student majoring in TR does an internship, the supervisor must expose the student to ___ of the task areas in the NCTRC Job Analysis.**

    a.  all

    b.  most

    c.  some

    d.  none

# Answer Key and Explanations

**1. C**: Mood (emotional state) and affect (the outward expression of the emotional state) are evaluated as part of psychosocial assessment.

- Flat affect: shows no facial expression.
- Broad affect: shows a wide range of facial and emotional expressions.
- Blunted affect: shows little facial expression or is very slow to show expressions.
- Inappropriate affect: shows a range of expressions, but they are inconsistent with mood or situation, especially inappropriate laughter or crying.
- Restricted affect: shows one type of expression regardless of circumstances.

**2. C**: Reduced cost of care is not an essential outcome although this may be a secondary benefit. Essential outcomes include improved physical health, reduced complications, and improved skills in coping with hospitalization. Other outcomes include improved healing, prevention of developmental delays, and improved family coping. Therapy for children is usually provided in hospitals and may involve individual or group play activities that help children adapt and understand treatments as well as restoring or maintaining function.

**3. D**: Havighurst's middle-age tasks include achieving civic and social responsibility, maintaining an economic standard of living, raising teenagers and teaching them to be responsible adults, developing leisure activity, accepting physiological changes related to aging and adjusting to aging of parents. Early adulthood tasks include finding a mate, marrying, having children, managing a home, getting started in an occupation or profession, assuming civic responsibility, and finding a congenial social group. Older adulthood tasks include adjusting to decreased physical strength and health, death of spouse, life in retirement, and reduced income; establishing ties with those in the same age group; meeting social and civic obligations; and establishing satisfactory physical living arrangements.

**4. A**: The most important consideration when choosing a recreational activity for a client is the client's interests. Asking the client what he/she likes to do and wants to do is the first step in engaging the client in therapy. While physical abilities and mental status are also important considerations, the goal of recreational therapy is to find innovative and creative ways to allow individuals to do those things that they enjoy. Costs must sometimes be considered as well.

**5. C**: Simulating playing with a hula-hoop improves balance and coordination. Video game sport simulators use a motion sensor to note body movement and control the game, so the client must stand upright and move the body to maintain momentum. Another useful activity is walking a tightrope. This gaming system is used in occupational, physical, and recreational therapy. One advantage to these video game simulators is that it allows clients to engage in virtual activities even before they are able to do so in reality.

**6. C**: Family Systems Theory states members of a family have different roles and behavioral patterns, so a change in one person's behavior will affect the others in the family. Health Belief Model predicts health behavior with the understanding that people take a health action to avoid negative consequences if the person expects that the negative outcome can be avoided and that he/she is able to do the action. Theory of Reasoned Action states the actions people take voluntarily can be predicted according to their personal attitude toward the action and their perception of how others will view the action. Theory of Planned Behavior evolved from the Theory of Reasoned Action when studies showed behavioral intention does not necessarily result in action.

**7. D**: Taking a CPR course is usually required for employment and cannot be counted for continuing education credit. Acceptable activities include attending continuing education courses, conferences, and workshops; taking academic courses; publishing articles; making conference presentations (including poster presentations); and completing professional work experience. The CTRS credential must be recertified every five years. Recertification requires 50 hours of continuing educations and 480 total hours of work over the five-year period in the recreation therapy profession.

**8. B**: The second principle of ATRA's Code of Ethics is nonmaleficence, which requires that the therapist use skills to assist clients while respecting the clients' rights to make decisions and preventing harm. The 10 principles (in order) include beneficence (maximizing benefits to clients), nonmaleficence, autonomy (right to choose), justice (fairness and equality), fidelity (meeting obligations), veracity (truth and honesty), informed consent, confidentiality and privacy (not disclosing protected information to third parties, competence (remaining current in education and skills), and compliance with laws and regulations.

**9. C**: OBRA (1987) requires that clients in nursing homes be engaged in a program of activities, which may include large group activities (singing, outings, fitness exercises), small group activities, and individualized outcome-focused activities. OAA (1965, rev. 2006) provides improved access to services for older adults and Native Americans. Provisions include the right of older Americans to participate in recreation activities as part of community care. ADA (1992) is civil rights legislation that provides the disabled, including those with mental impairment, access to employment and the community. HIPAA (1996) addresses the rights of the individual related to portability and privacy of health information.

**10. D**: Telling family members that a client states he is depressed is a violation of HIPAA regulations related to privacy of information and is not an example of client advocacy. Encouraging the client to discuss his feelings with family members is more effective and protects the clients right to confidentiality. Advocacy may start with simply listening to the client and observing the client for fears, apprehensions, conflicts, or concerns that may impede progress. Team members need to be aware of observable problems, such as apprehensions, that may affect the plan of care. Advocacy may include directly intervening or requesting interventions to meet client needs.

**11. B**: Beep baseball, which uses special balls that beep and padded upright cylinders that buzz at bases to help guide the runners, was designed for the vision impaired. Each team has a pitcher and catcher who are sighted. The rules of beep baseball are somewhat different from standard baseball. The pitcher announces each pitch and tries to aim at the player's bat. The National Beep Baseball Association (NBBA) has established rules for the games and can provide information for those wanting to establish a beep baseball team.

**12. A**: Kolb's Model of Experiential Learning is based on acquiring knowledge through grasping experience and transforming that experience into knowledge through cognitive processes and perception. Experience may be transformed into knowledge through abstract conceptualizing (analyzing, thinking), observing others, or actively experimenting. This model stresses that the individual makes choices between the concrete and the abstract, and this is reflected in learning styles.

- Diverging: concrete experience and reflective observation
- Assimilating: abstract conceptualization and reflective observation
- Converging: abstract conceptualization and active experimentation
- Accommodating: concrete experience and reflective observation

**13. C**: The best solution for a client is always the one that allows for the most functional independence, so providing a clip-on plate edge helps prevent the client pushing food from the plate. Non-skid plate mats are placed under plates to prevent them from sliding off of the table when the person is eating. Clients should not have diet limited to liquids or finger foods if they are able to eat a regular diet. Assisting the client should be limited to that which is necessary, and feeding the client should be a last resort as it makes the client completely dependent in eating.

**14. B**: Piaget's preoperational stage (ages 2-7 years) comprises the preconceptual substage (ages 2-4 years), in which children use language and symbols but have poor logical ability and show egocentrism; and the intuitive substage (ages 4-7 years), in which children establish a concept of cause and effect, which may be faulty because of transductive reasoning. They may engage in magical thinking, centration, and animism. Stages in order include:

- Sensorimotor (ages 0-24 months): gain motor skills, show affects, behave with intention, gain spatial awareness, and begin use of language.
- Preoperational (ages 2-7 years).
- Concrete Operational (ages 7-11 years): better understand cause and effect, concrete objects, and conservation.
- Formal Operational (11-adult): acquire mature thought processes and the ability to think abstractly.

**15. D**: Clients with tactile sensitivity usually dislike activities related to grooming, such as washing or brushing hair or brushing teeth. Other indications include hypersensitivity related to different textures and avoidance of those that are rough or irritating. They may prefer certain clothing, such as a soft sweatshirt, and avoid others, such as heavy jeans or clothes with appliqués or labels that touch the skin. They may avoid going barefoot and get upset if their hands, face, or clothing are dirty. They may have excessive reactions to painful stimuli.

**16. A**: Pseudohypertrophic (Duchenne) muscular dystrophy is characterized by enlargement of muscles by fatty infiltration associated with muscular atrophy, which causes contractures and deformities of joints. Abnormal bone development results in spinal and other skeletal deformities. The disease progresses rapidly, and most children are wheelchair bound by about 12 years of age. Other types include:

- Facioscapulohumeral (ages 10-24 years): weakness in the upper arms, shoulders angled forward, and a lack of facial mobility.
- Limb Girdle (age varies from late childhood to middle age): weakness of proximal muscles of the pelvic and shoulder girdles.
- Oculopharyngeal (ages 40-70 years): weakness of eyelid muscles and throat muscles.

**17. B**: Discontinuing all self-contained special programs is not characteristic of (or necessary for) placing a child in the least restrictive environment as these programs may provide benefit. For example, a child with autistic disorder may receive special training is a self-contained program but still be placed in an environment as close to traditional as possible for most activities. Children should be placed according to individual needs rather than placed by diagnosis (group placement) alone. Providing alternatives shows respect for the individual by allowing some autonomy.

**18. A**: Assisting the man to take the bus independently to enjoy leisure activities, such as attending a movie theater, is an example of normalization because he is participating in normal adult activities with support. Placement in a long-term care facility is not a normal situation although some normalization may be possible. While the individual may be guided in choosing more age-appropriate choices, refusing to allow him to play with children's toys is coercive and does not show respect for his autonomy. Practice and guidance in how to behave in different situations may be part of working toward normalization, but expecting him to follow "rules" is too directive.

**19. C**: The first step in ensuring that inclusion is successful is to assess the individual needs of each adolescent. Once needs are identified, the 3 other critical elements are to identify a source of funding, identify support staff, and provide training. If possible, support staff should be in the same age range as the participants so that they can feel more independent, but this may vary according to need. Some adolescent may require constant support while others may have minimal needs. Training should include methods of adapting activities and dealing with behavioral differences.

**20. D**: The bowling ramp is the most appropriate intervention because it allows the woman to bowl by placing the ball at the top of the sloped ramp rather than swinging and throwing the ball. The Bradshaw Bowl Buggy is a wheelchair especially designed for bowling, but this client is not wheelchair bound. Because her balance and mobility are poor, a modified bowling ball with a grip handle or bowling ball pusher would not be safe for her, as she would be at risk for falls.

**21. C**: IDEA does not guarantee a disabled child the best available education. Provisions include free public appropriate public education provided according to an individualized education program (IEP) in the least restrictive environment. The IEP is developed with the parents, regular and special education teachers, school psychologist or other person who can evaluate child's needs, and an administrator or other person with authority to make decisions about the child's education. Children with disabilities are also covered by ADA, but the same modifications can be provided under IDEA based on the IEP. ALL disabled children qualify for educational services (zero reject rule), even if they appear unable to benefit.

**22. B**: Agitation and combative behavior is often a sign of fear or discomfort in a person with dementia, so the first step is to analyze the pattern of agitation to try to determine the cause. Agitation may be related to needs, such as thirst, hunger, or need to urinate or defecate, or it may be related to certain activities or people. Once the pattern is identified, then steps to alleviate the trigger can be developed. CTRSs may need to try various approaches to alleviating the person's distress, evaluating each approach for effectiveness. Restraints should be avoided as they increase agitation.

**23. A**: Changes in personality, impulsive risk-taking behavior, and little facial emotion are consistent with traumatic injury to a frontal lobe, which controls personality and emotions. Damage to the right frontal lobe may result in pseudopsychopathic behavior and damage to the left in pseudodepression. Fine motor dysfunction of the upper extremities may occur as well. Divergent thinking, which includes problem solving, may be impaired. The left frontal lobe is associated with language (in most people), and damage here may result in Broca's aphasia.

**24. D**: A speech disorder is not a specific characteristic of ADHD although associated learning problems may impact language development and patterns of speech. ADHD is characterized by inattention, including poor concentration, difficulty paying attention and staying on task, poor planning, inability to monitor behavior, and difficulty learning new material. Hyperactivity signs include restlessness, constant movement, and changing activities. Impulsivity is evident by the person's acting out before thinking.

**25. C**: Security is always a concern in a correctional facility, and staff is not permitted to divulge personal information. The best response is "I'm sorry. I can't discuss personal information" as this is factual and shows more respect for the individual than giving an order, such as "Don't ask personal questions" or questioning the inmate. The CTRS can be friendly and supportive of inmates, encouraging participation, but should avoid becoming friends or sharing personal information even though it may seem harmless.

**26. B**: A doll demonstration is probably the best teaching tool for a 32-month-old child who is deaf or hearing-impaired. The CTRS can begin with the demonstration and encourage the child to play with the doll, guiding the child to put the doll through the same activities and moving on to having the child do the activities as part of play. Video and pictures may be helpful for older children who can better focus attention, but young children often do better when they can learn through play. A child of this age probably knows minimal sign language, so a sign language interpreter is not needed.

**27. D**: Conflict resolution should begin by allowing both sides to present their side of the conflict without bias, focusing on opinions rather than individuals. Other steps (not necessarily in order) include:

- Encouraging cooperation through negotiation and compromise.
- Providing guidance to keep the discussions on track and avoid arguments.
- Evaluating the need for renegotiation, formal resolution process, or a third party.
- Utilizing humor and empathy to defuse escalating tensions.
- Summarizing the issues and outlining key arguments.
- Avoiding a forced resolution, if possible.

**28. D**: FIM scores range from 18 (total dependence) to 126 (total independence), and a score of 63 comprised of 3 or 4 in each of 18 categories suggests the need for minimal to moderate contact assistance. The client will require an aide to assist with ambulation and other activities. Lower FIM scores on admission correlate with longer need for in-client rehabilitation. FIM scores are included as part of the Inpatient Rehabilitation Facility Client Assessment Instrument required by Medicare for reimbursement for care.

**29. C**: According to Knowles, adult learners tend to be practical and goal-oriented, so they like to remain organized and keep the goal in mind while learning. Adult learners also tend to be:

- Self-Directed: Adults like active involvement and responsibility.
- Knowledgeable: Adults can relate new material to information with which they are familiar through life experience or education.
- Relevancy-Oriented: Adults like to know how they will use information.
- Motivated: Adults like to see evidence of their own achievement, such as by gaining a certificate.

**30. B**: All staff members are responsible for identifying performance improvement projects. Performance improvement must be a continuous process. Continuous quality improvement (CQI) is a management philosophy that emphasizes the organization and systems and processes within that organization rather than individuals. Total quality management (TQM) is a management philosophy that espouses a commitment to meeting the needs of the customers (clients and staff) at all levels within an organization. Both management philosophies recognize that change can be made in small steps and should involve staff at all levels.

**31. A**: The primary purpose of supervision is promoting the intern's professional growth and development of skills while still protecting the integrity of the program. Supervision is also part of mentoring and provides opportunities for problem solving, especially if errors are identified or the intern is using incorrect practices. Supervisors should focus on both strengths and weaknesses. Supervisors should be experienced and knowledgeable about current best practices. While information gleaned from supervision may be part of the basis for grading the intern, this is not the primary purpose.

**32. B**: The treatment plan is documented in the planning stage. Different documentation is done for each phase.

- Assessment: Observe and question. Document leisure activities and usual activities prior to treatment admissions form.
- Planning: Based on assessment, document plan of care, including frequency of therapy and short-term and long-term goals.
- Implementation: Document progress notes.
- Evaluation: Document discharge plan, including achievement of goals or reasons goals were not achieved, such as medical setbacks.

**33. A**: Observing the client doing arts and crafts projects provides the best opportunity to evaluate the client's ability to stay on task and concentrate because these projects usually require the ability to organize, solve problems, and carry out a number of sequential steps. Personal reading is more difficult to evaluate without testing the person because people can appear to be actively reading when they are not processing what they are reading. Treadmill walking is a physical activity that requires little concentration or problem solving.

**34. A**: Subjective notes usually quote what the client states directly: "I can't exercise. My foot hurts." Objective notes record clinical facts that are observed: Client limping and avoiding pressure on left foot so is unable to participate in dancing activity. Blister noted on left heel. Assessment relates to evaluation of subjective and objective notes: Poorly fitted shoes causing friction rub and blisters. Plan is based on assessment: Treat and protect blisters. Obtain properly fitted shoes.

**35. D**: Carol Peterson's Leisure Ability Model, which aims to develop an appropriate leisure lifestyle for all clients, comprises three primary components.

- Treatment is geared toward assessing disability and improving function so that clients are able to engage in leisure activities.
- Leisure education focuses on the knowledge, skills, and abilities the client needs to engage in activities.
- Recreation participation provides opportunities, usually structured, for clients to engage in leisure activities. Under this model, activities that the client does outside of structured environments are also considered part of recreation therapy.

**36. A**: The utilitarian ethical approach is to select that activity that provides the most good for the most people, so it focuses on the majority. In this case, the sing-along could provide participation or enjoyment for the majority of people while people with cognizant or physical impairment may not be able to participate in Monopoly or video game simulated sports competition. People who are bed bound or wheelchair bound probably couldn't participate in the outdoor walk. Taking people on the walk in wheelchairs may be staff-intensive. One problem with the utilitarian approach is the needs of the minority are overlooked.

**37. A**: Ethical principles concerning client confidentiality prevent the CTRS from divulging private information, and this covers statements about feelings or intent, such as "I hate my father. I wish he were dead." While this may be cause for concern and should prompt further discussion, there is no inherent threat of harm to another individual or to the client. While there is not complete consensus, most ethicists agree that confidentiality may be violated only in instances where clients pose a threat to themselves (cutting or overdose) or others (injury or murder).

**38. D**: A pre-transfer assessment should review physical, cognitive, and emotional statuses and determine the client's level of independence and functional skills.

- Physical: body weight; knee, shoulder, and arm extension; presence of muscle spasms; balance (lateral and anterior-posterior); mobility; need for assistive devices; weight-bearing ability; and upper-body strength.
- Cognitive: ability to communicate and understand, and awareness of safety issues.
- Emotional: motivation, fears, and concerns.

**39. C**: Transferring a client from a wheelchair that is not on level ground may result in the chair tipping, which increases the risk of falls or injury, so the car and wheelchair should move to a level area. It's easier to navigate an area that is not level than to transfer from it. Using two people for transfer and braking and blocking the wheels will not prevent tipping. Attempting to level the wheels may pose additional risks to the client.

**40. D**: Feedback should be contingent, motivational, and informational. If a client is successful, feedback will be primarily contingent and motivational, but if the client is unsuccessful, feedback may focus more on contingent and informational.

- Contingent: Acknowledge the effort the person makes; for example, "Try that one more time," "It's hard to get this right at first," or "Watch me while I demonstrate." Avoid directly negative statements such as, "You're not doing this right."
- Motivational: Provide positive feedback and through words, such as, "Good try," and expressions, like smiling and head nodding.
- Informational: Provide specific information necessary to do task or to correct errors; for example, "Move your right foot forward."

**41. B**: Acknowledging what the client actually does—"You used good problem-solving skills"—is the best response because it focuses on the person and action rather than the disability. Ascribing clients with disabilities as "brave" when they are doing daily activities, even those related to falls, or overly empathizing with "I'm so sorry" may be interpreted as patronizing. Suggesting the client should have called for help is putting him in a dependent position and failing to recognize his autonomy.

**42. B**: Passive-aggressive behavior is common in those who have difficulty asserting themselves, so a referral for assertiveness training may benefit this client. Clients often become angry and frustrated because their wants and needs are not recognized, but they lack the skills to assert themselves in a positive manner. Assertiveness training often includes role-playing, feedback, and exercises that help the client learn new types of social interpersonal skills. Being assertive allows the client to express directly what he or she wants rather than trying to effect change through passive-aggressive behavior.

**43. C**: Industry vs inferiority, according to Erikson's Psychosocial Development Model.

- Trust vs mistrust (birth to 1 year old): mistrust or faith and optimism.
- Autonomy vs shame/doubt (1-3 years old): doubt and shame or self-control and willpower.
- Initiative vs guilt (3-6 years old): guilt or direction and purpose.
- Industry vs inferiority (6-12 years): inadequacy and inferiority or competence.
- Identify vs role confusion (12-18 years): role confusion or devotion and fidelity to others.
- Intimacy vs isolation (young adulthood): lack of close relationships or love and intimacy.
- Generativity vs stagnation (middle age): stagnation or caring and achievements.
- Ego integrity vs despair (older adulthood): despair (failure to accept changes of aging) or wisdom (acceptance).

**44. A**: Shakiness, diarrhea, and agitation are early signs of mild to moderate lithium toxicity. Other symptoms include increased thirst and increased frequency of urination as well as general muscle weakness and impaired coordination. Seizures and lack of consciousness are signs of more severe lithium toxicity. Lithium, a mood stabilizer, is used primarily for the treatment of bipolar disease because it controls mood swings, especially by preventing episodes of manic behavior. Clients taking lithium should have regular blood tests to ensure levels are within therapeutic range.

**45. D**: In the leaning side-to-side pressure release, weight should be taken completely off of one buttock for 30 to 90 seconds before returning to neutral position and then leaning to the other side. The duration depends on a number of variables, including the person's size and weight, duration of sitting, and time period since last pressure release. Alternately, the client may lean forward with the chest touching the knees or grip the armrests to lift the body away from the chair.

**46. A**: Raynaud's syndrome results in intermittent arterial vasoconstriction of the hands and/or feet, nose, and ears, especially in response to cold or stress, so clients should exercise in a warm environment. Exercising in the cold, even when wearing gloves and multiple layers of clothing, may trigger an episode in which the affected parts become very pale (white) then cyanotic (blue) and cold followed by a recovery phase in which the area appears flushed (red). Clients should be encouraged to exercise regularly. Relaxation exercises may help to relieve symptoms.

**47. B**: Sweating, flushing above the level of injury, severe headache, nasal congestion, anxiety, and nausea are consistent with autonomic dysreflexia, which occurs with central cord lesions at or above T6 when a painful stimulus occurs below the spinal cord injury. Autonomic dysreflexia occurs only after the initial spinal shock has resolved. Onset is often very sudden and constitutes a medical emergency. Common causes include distended bladder, fecal impaction, pressure sores, tight clothing, hyperthermia, and other painful stimuli. The first response is to do a pressure release and loosen clothing. If initial actions are unsuccessful, the client should be examined for bladder distention and/or constipation or fecal impaction.

**48. C**: Conditioned play audiometry (CPA) is appropriate for children 2-5 years of age. Screening methods vary according to age.

- 0 to 6 months: otoacoustic emissions (OAE) or auditory brainstem response (ABR).
- 6 to 24 months: visual reinforcement audiometry (VRA). The child is rewarded with visual reinforcement, such as a moving toy or light, when looking toward a sound source.

- 2 to 5 years: conditioned play audiometry (CPA). The child is provided a demonstration and taught to do a particular activity, like putting a block in a box, each time the child hears a sound.
- 5 years onward: standard audiometry. The child indicates by various methods, such as raising hand or pushing a buzzer, when a sound is heard.

**49. A**: Van Andel, Carter, and Robb's Therapeutic Recreation Service Delivery Model's scope of practice includes four components.

- Diagnosis/needs and assessment includes field observation, standardized tests, and other assessments.
- Treatment/rehabilitation includes prescriptive recreational activities to stabilize or restore functioning and health.
- Education includes cognitive exercises, leisure education, skills training, and any education that aids the client's ability to function.
- Prevention/health promotion includes stress management, smoking cessation, and exercise programs to help promote health and prevent loss of function.
- Initially, the client provides informed consent, but therapy is directed by the CTRS with a goal of client independence and self-sufficiency at the end of treatment.

**50. C**: A good strategy for helping a client overcome feelings of low self-esteem includes providing opportunities for the client to make decisions. Other strategies include providing companionship, listening, and encouraging the client to express her feelings and concerns. Positive feedback and praise should be given when earned rather than praising everything. Telling the client that she has no reason to be depressed will invalidate her feelings and further lower her self-esteem. Low self-esteem is common among older adults because they have to deal with so many losses. They may become depressed, passive, and dependent.

**51. A**: The best method to evaluate a client's educational outcomes after teaching a procedure is to ask the client to do a demonstration. Client feedback isn't a reliable indicator of ability to perform. Tests, whether oral or written, can identify what a client knows and may be appropriate for testing general knowledge about a subject, such as diet, but knowing and doing are different skills, so demonstration is critical and allows the CTRS to provide feedback or additional training if needed.

**52. C**: The timed-up-and-go (TUG) test assesses mobility and the risk of falls. The patient sits in a chair with armrests, stands, walks three meters, and turns and sits back down. Normal time is 7 to 10 seconds. Those requiring more than 14 seconds are at risk for falls. The TUG-cognitive, a modified version, requires the person to carry out the test while counting backwards from a number between 20 and 100. The TUG-manual version requires the person to carry out the test while carrying a cup full of water. The longer the time required for these tasks, the higher the risk and the lower the functional ability.

**53. D**: Computer terminals must be placed where others cannot read notes being written, and access must be password protected. These systems may include clinical decision support systems (CDSS), which provide diagnosis and treatment options based on symptoms. Terminals are often placed at point of care but may be located elsewhere, such as at unit stations; easy access and comfortable height are important. Computerized charting is legible, tamper-proof, and tends to reduce errors as many systems signal if a treatment is missed or the wrong treatment is given.

**54. C**: Schizophrenia is characterized by personality disintegration and distortion in the perception of reality, thought processes, and social development, including delusions, withdrawal, odd behavior, hallucinations, inability to care for oneself, disorganized speech, catatonia, alogia (inability to speak), mental confusion, aphasia, hearing voices, and avolition. Major depressive disorder is characterized by depressed mood, a profound and constant sense of hopelessness and despair, and a loss of interest in all or almost all activities. Bipolar disorder is characterized by mood swings that may include mania, depression, or both. Narcissistic personality disorder is characterized by a heightened feeling of self-importance, persistent patterns of grandiosity, a need for admiration, disregard for other people's rights, restraint in expression of feelings, and a lack of empathy.

**55. D**: People with addictive behavior typically try to hide their addiction. They do not have the ability to control the extent of their addiction and cannot stop using. Signs include obsession with acquiring addictive substances, compulsive use of substances, denial of addiction, as well as experiencing blackouts, episodes of depression, and withdrawal on cessation of drug use. People may lie or steal in order to acquire addictive substances. Even after cessation of use, addicts frequently crave addictive substances and may relapse if they do not have an adequate support system, such as Alcoholics Anonymous or Narcotics Anonymous.

**56. A**: Prescriptive play therapy is used primarily to treat specific symptoms or behavioral problems. The CTRS assesses the needs of the individual child and selects particular interventions based on literature review and experience. Filial therapy is a child-centered structured therapy that includes training parents and then observing them in play sessions with the child and providing feedback in order to improve family dynamics. Theraplay aims to improve attachment between parent and child through adult-supervised interactive play and to increase the child's trust and self-esteem. Core concepts include structure, engagement, nurture, and challenge. Cognitive behavioral play therapy focuses on helping the child make behavioral changes by learning new strategies and receiving support.

**57. B**: Compensation theory states that people tend to engage in leisure activities that are different from their work experience. Spillover theory states that people tend to engage in leisure activities that are an extension of, or similar to, the type of work they are engaged in. Relaxation therapy states that the primary goal of leisure activity is relaxation and stress reduction. Generalization theory states that people transfer rewarded behaviors to leisure, so they pick leisure activities in which they can use similar skills and behavior.

**58. B**: Anorexia and weight loss associated with topiramate may exacerbate the patient's tendency toward anorexia. Sedation may occur initially but usually subsides. Dulling of cognition may occur, but starting with a low dose and increasing gradually may avoid this effect. Many other anticonvulsants are associated with weight gain and increased appetite, and this is sometimes a concern for adolescents. Generalized tonic-clonic seizures can occur at any age and usually have abrupt onset with loss of consciousness for one to two minutes. Seizures may include drooling, eyes rolling upward or deviating to one side, and urinary or bowel incontinence.

**59. C**: The first step in an activity task analysis is to determine the tasks the client does or needs to do as well as when, where, and how the activity is carried out. Then, the activity is divided into component parts so that the clients can master a small part of the activity at a time. The CTRS may create a flow chart, outline, or checklist to guide therapy. The CTRS devises different strategies to help the client master each step in the activity and identifies the desired outcomes.

**60. D**: Preferred Provider Organization (PPO) provides discounted rates for those on Medicare who choose healthcare providers from a list of those who have agreed to accept Medicare assignment. Medicare Managed Care is provided by a health maintenance organization (HMO), which receives payment for services rather than the traditional pay-for-service Medicare payment system. Prospective Payment System (PPS) pays a set amount for patient care, depending upon diagnosis (diagnosis-related group or DRG). Private insurance pay-for-service Medicare plans are contracted by Medicare and may provide more benefits, but the patient may be required to work individually with the insurance company to determine benefits and may be assessed an additional monthly fee.

**61. D**: Socioeconomic barriers, such as lack of job and insurance, are probably the primary obstacles to care. The very poor may have access to free programs or Medicaid, but middle-class workers, such as a nurse, may be ineligible for assistance. Other barriers include

- Organizational: inadequate wheelchair access, waiting lists, and a lack of interpreters.
- Geographic: lack of local facilities or CTRSs, especially in economically depressed inner-city and rural areas.
- Linguistic: inability to speak or understand enough English to communicate needs and concerns.
- Cultural: lack of understanding about therapy, different health beliefs, and bias.

**62. A**: A high check-in counter presents a barrier to clients who are short or wheelchair bound. Many elements are included in an accessible environment, such as compliance with all ADA requirements for universal access. Accessibility is enhanced by adjustable chairs; light and sound alarm systems; sensitivity training regarding disabilities, different cultures, and genders; sitting and standing scales; TTY availability; interpreter availability; signs with Braille and/or raised lettering; and power-door operations.

**63. B**: The correct procedure to assisting a visually impaired client is to offer an arm so the client is guided rather than led. Using a wheelchair is not appropriate if the client is ambulatory unless a wheelchair is required by facility regulations or the client requests use of a wheelchair. The CTRS should always strive toward normalization when assisting a client with any type of disability, allowing the client to be as independent as possible. The CTRS should speak normally and describe the route or barriers, such as "We're approaching a door."

**64. B**: A telephone interview of a friend and neighbor is not an appropriate source of assessment data because HIPAA precludes providing any information about a client—even that fact that the person is a client. Care must always be taken to avoid breaching confidentiality. However, the husband is part of the client's support system and may provide valuable information. Other sources of information include copies of hospital records, laboratory reports, discharge summaries, social worker reports, and staff reports.

**65. A**: Because diabetes is associated with circulatory impairment, even a small sore may develop into a larger ulcer and gangrene, so the client should be advised to see a physician immediately. Loose protective gauze dressing may be applied and the client advised to wear a soft slipper to prevent further irritation until the client sees the physician. Shoes should be checked to make sure they are properly fitted, but the sore may have developed from other injuries, such as going barefoot and stubbing the toe.

**66. C**: COPD is associated with air trapping, so clients have limited air exchange; thus, the goal is to increase the inspiration/expiration ratio to 1:2 so that expirations are prolonged and a greater volume of air is exhaled. Exercises should incorporate diaphragmatic breathing and pursed lip breathing. The primary components of COPD include:

- Progressive airflow limitation.
- Inflammatory response that causes a narrowing of the peripheral airways and a thickening of the vessel walls of the pulmonary vasculature.
- Exertional dyspnea and chronic cough.

**67. B**: Standard precautions are used with clients who are HIV positive, so gloves should be worn for contact with bodily fluids, including blood, urine, feces, or saliva, or skin that is not intact due to rash or sores. Personal protective equipment (PPE), such as a gown, a mask, or goggles, is only necessary if there is a possibility that fluids may splash on the clothes or face. Hand hygiene (washing, alcohol rub) should be practiced before and after working with the client.

**68. D**: The Public Health Model focuses on achieving good health and a sense of wellbeing as a basic right of human beings and proposes that opportunities (diagnosis/treatment) to achieve this should be available to all groups. The Medical Model focuses on the individual and pathology and includes identification of underlying disorder, interventions, treatments, and cures. The Psychosocial Rehabilitation Model focuses on restoring those with mental disorders to the community as functioning society members with a sense of wellbeing. The Community Model focuses on steps that communities can take to develop preventive programs to effect change.

**69. D**: Social psychological carrying capacity refers to the maximum number of people and interactions that can occur before they negatively impact participants. This is the effect people have on other people. Thus, when planning activities, the CTRS must determine the point at which overload may occur in terms of people, noise, confusion, and interactions, preventing people from benefiting from the activity. Biological carrying capacity is the maximum use/stress/activity an organism can withstand before deterioration or damage occurs. Use density refers to the number of people in a given space.

**70. C**: This refers to the norming stage. Tuckman's model includes four stages.

- Forming: During the team-building stage, people try to avoid conflict and want to be accepted. They begin to assess the group and gather information.
- Storming: Conflicts arise and can doom the group to failure without guidance toward compromise.
- Norming: People develop a sense of trust and are able to communicate ideas and make progress toward an agreed-upon goal.
- Performing: Team members are able to carry out cooperative action to attain goals.

**71. B**: While the CTRS's concern is for the comfort of the clients, the assessment is based on stereotyping, making assumptions about an individual based on ideas about a group. While one can say that the Hispanic culture and Chinese culture as a whole are different, one can never make that assumption about individuals in those cultures. Additionally, people from different cultures often work together well. Prejudice is a negative opinion about someone based simply on that person's race, gender, or religion. Bias is a preference for one over another. Discrimination is unfair treatment of someone based on personal prejudice.

**72. A**: Because this is a relatively small group with limited time, the best approach is to develop group activities with individual accommodations so that the group is all focused on similar projects but with different approaches according to their abilities. For example, if working on fine arts, such as painting, some people may paint pictures of scenes or items while others paint abstract designs with color. Some may use acrylic paints or watercolors while others use colored marking pens. Focusing on one type of activity encourages group interaction, positive feedback, and a sense of belonging.

**73. A**: Adapted swimming lessons for children with disabilities is an example of a therapeutic recreation leisure service because the goal is primarily to allow children to participate in a leisure activity. Swimming classes that focus on increasing muscle strength would be a health service, as are balance exercises for stroke patients. Classes to teach skills, such as social skills and microwave cooking, are educational services, as they teach people how to accommodate their disabilities and remain engaged in normal activities.

**74. B**: The occupational therapist's primary focus is on helping clients manage activities of daily living, such as dressing, bathing, and preparing food. The rehabilitation therapist devises methods to assist clients to return to normal physical, mental, and emotional functioning. The physical therapist uses special equipment and exercises to help people regain or maintain body strength and physical function. The psychologist provides research, testing and assessment, and therapy for psychological or behavioral disorders.

**75. B**: A capital budget determines which capital projects (such as remodeling, repairing, or purchasing of equipment or buildings) will be allocated funding for the year. These capital expenditures are usually based on a cost-benefit analysis and prioritization of needs. An operating budget is used for daily operations and includes general expenses, such as salaries, education, insurance, maintenance, depreciation, debts, and profit. The budget has three elements: statistics, expenses, and revenue. A cash balance budget projects cash balances for a specific future time period, including all operating and capital budget items. A master budget combines operating, capital, and cash balance budgets as well as any specialized or area-specific budgets.

**76. A**: Bureaucratic: follows organization rules exactly and expects everyone else to do so. Autocratic: makes decisions independently, and strictly enforces rules. Democratic: presents a problem and asks staff or teams to arrive at a solution, although the leader usually makes the final decision. Charismatic: depends upon personal charisma to influence people, and may be very persuasive but may engage "followers" and relate to one group rather than the organization. Laissez-faire: exerts little direct control but allows employees or teams to make decisions with little interference. Consultative: presents a decision and welcomes input and questions although decisions rarely change. Participatory: presents a potential decision and makes final decision based on input from staff or teams.

**77. A**: The primary goal of risk management is to identify potential risks and provide plans to reduce risks, so risk management is proactive as well as reactive in that risk management also manages problems that arise. Risks may relate to client safety as well as financial risks. A written risk management plan should include specific and measurable goals and policies, such as those regarding confidentiality and conflict of interest, and should clarify the responsibility for reporting and both the method and frequency of evaluation. Essential tasks of risk management include educating staff about methods to reduce risk and documenting accountability.

**78. B**: A Mini-Cog test assesses dementia by having patients remember and repeat three common objects and draw a clock face indicating a particular time. The Mini-Mental State Examination (MMSE) assesses dementia through a series of tests, including remembering the names of three common objects, counting backward, naming, providing location, copying shapes, and following directions. The Digit Repetition Test assesses attention by asking the patient to repeat two numbers, then three, then four, and so on. The Confusion Assessment Method is used to assess delirium, not dementia.

**79. B**: David Austin's Health Improvement/Health Promotion (HI/HP) model is based on the premise that the stability tendency lessens as a client gains optimal health and moves toward actualization. The HI/HP model aims to help clients recover from health threats and obtain optimal health through prescriptive activities, recreation, and leisure activities. Health protection is prescriptive and exemplified by the stabilizing tendency that pushes clients to achieve health. During this stage, clients have little choice and the CTRS directs activities. During the recreation phase, the client has more control and moves away from stability tendency toward actualization tendency and finally to client-directed leisure and actualization.

**80. D**: Because objectives are the means by which a goal is met, they must be measurable: walking for 30 minutes, five times a week. Using terms such as "regularly," "weekly," or "daily" is less clear as the duration is not delineated. Signing up for a class doesn't mean that the person attends or participates. Making specific measurable objectives also provides a target for the client to work toward and a basis for evaluation of compliance. The CTRS should assure that all activities for the client are goal-directed with measurable objectives.

**81. D**: Inclusion recreation includes programs and activities for both disabled and non-disabled children. Training staff and providing support and some accommodations allow disabled children to participate fully and to learn valuable social and leisure skills. Programs are essentially enhanced without major changes. Disabled children are assessed to determine their need for accommodations. This assessment includes determining their interest in recreation (including indoor and outdoor activities, community involvement, travel, and hobbies), degree of social functioning (ability to follow directions, sit quietly, and interact with others), medications, specific disability, ability to communicate and method of communication (speech, sign language, or assistive device), feeding and eating skills, mobility, and toileting skills.

**82. C**: A dual relationship is one in which the CTRS has a relationship with the client outside of the therapeutic environment. Because dual relationships can result in conflict, the client should be reassigned. A conflict of interest occurs when self-interest interferes with the CTRS carrying out a professional role. A boundary violation occurs when the boundary between the professional role of the CTRS and the client is breached, such as engaging in sexual behavior, giving or receiving gifts, coercing, providing extra attention, and sharing personal information. Confidentiality, keeping personal information private, can be maintained, as the exact nature of the dual relationship does not need to be outlined.

**83. B**: Reliability is scoring consistency with different CTRSs. Validity is the ability to measure as intended; for example, tests to measure function possess validity if they actually measure function. Fairness is the absence of bias regarding gender, education, race, etc., that skews the results. Staff preference may be based on ease of use or familiarity, so preference alone is not a good indicator. Practicality requires consideration of multiple issues, such as cost, staff training, space, and necessary materials. Availability is whether or not the assessment can be used or obtained when needed.

**84. C**: The ASIA (American Spinal Injury Association) impairment scale is used to classify the degree of spinal cord injury and the strength of 10 key muscles, graded on a scale from 0 (complete paralysis) to 5 (active movement against resistance). Spinal injuries are classified on a scale from A to E.

- Complete injury to the spinal cord with no sensory or motor function.
- Incomplete injury with sensory but no motor function.
- Incomplete injury with motor function and more than 50% of muscles below injury are less than grade 3.
- Incomplete injury with motor function and more than 50% of muscles below injury are more than or equal to grade 3.
- Normal sensory and motor findings.

**85. D**: The Play Interaction Checklist is appropriate for ages 3 to 6 years. While the CTRS may respond to the children if approached, the CTRS should avoid engaging the children in conversation, as this will change the dynamics of social interaction. The child should be observed playing with a variety of toys with a group of familiar peers, if possible, because a child may act differently with children the child doesn't know. A series of two or more observations is more reliable than a single observation. The CTRS should observe other three-year-olds for comparison.

**86. C**: The Comprehensive Evaluation in Recreational Therapy (CERT)—Physical Disabilities tool assesses functions needed for leisure skills: gross and fine motor function and skills, communication, locomotion, sensory function, cognitive ability, and behavior. The Leisure Diagnostic Battery (LDB) tool has eight different components focusing on the client's perceptions regarding his or her leisure experience, including perceptions of leisure functioning, leisure freedom, barriers to leisure, and leisure preferences. The Leisure Motivation Scale (LMS) tool assesses four primary motivators to engaging in leisure activities: social, intellectual, competence-mastery, and stimulus avoidance. The Leisure Satisfaction Measure (LSM) tool assesses the client's perception of whether leisure is meeting his or her psychological, educational, social, physiological, and aesthetic needs.

**87. D**: Prescription is not within the scope of practice of the CTRS, which includes activities that promote optimal health and function and aim to help the client reduce limitations to full participation in community life. Elements of practice include assessing, planning, designing, and implementing programs; consulting; and engaging in research and educational projects that advocate for recreation therapy. The recreation therapist may work with groups or individuals that need recreation therapy or interventions to promote leisure activities.

**88. A**: The purpose of a functional vision assessment is to determine the ability to use vision to function and is usually conducted with children with impaired vision. This is an observational study. The child is observed doing a variety of tasks to determine how the child uses close vision (closer than 16 inches), intermediate vision (16-36 inches), and distant vision (more than 36 inches). Assessments include eye preference, hand-eye coordination, color discrimination, tracking, fixating, scanning, and shifting of gaze. The results are used to help select environmental modifications and adaptive devices.

**89. A**: A broad affect shows a wide range of expressions and is not consistent with depression, which is more commonly characterized by flat or blunted affect. Indications of depression or withdrawal include slumping, closed posture (sometimes with arms crossed), failure to make eye contact, and sitting with the body turned away from the interviewer. Other indications include tiredness or agitation and difficulty focusing on conversation or making decisions. The client may show no interest in the program and no motivation to participate.

**90. B**: The creation of the ATRA stemmed from the need and desire for a national organization that represented recreation therapists. The need for ATRA resulted from the dissatisfaction that recreation therapists felt in their representation by the NTRS. ATRA proponents would argue that the NTRS lacked a clear philosophical direction and mission due to the fact that they attempted to combine recreation therapists with the subdivision of parks and recreation from which NTRS as formed. For this reason, there were often differing opinions between those with a clinical background (recreation therapists) and those who simply wished to promote recreation among all without clinical basis (parks and recreation). Therefore, in 1984, ATRA was formed to represent the specific vision and needs of recreation therapists.

**91. D**: As described by Erikson and other theorists of lifespan human growth and development, toddlers begin to assert their need for autonomy as they learn to control their actions; and adolescents seek to separate from dependence on parents as they establish their own personal identities. Young adults (A) typically have resolved this issue more or less. Infants have not yet developed enough to be able to assert independence, and children in the early elementary years (B) are focused on new academic and social challenges more than autonomy. Erikson characterized middle adulthood as a time of generating a legacy for future generations, and old-age adulthood of life review (C).

**92. A**: In the "nature/nurture" debate, nature is a word to represent characteristics that are genetically inherited, while nurture represents characteristics that are environmentally learned. Genetics/heredity is not equal to personality, which includes both inherited and learned parts; and nurture does not equal behaviors (C), which are also both innate and learned. Nature concerns inborn traits, not neglect; and nurture concerns all acquired traits, not limited to education (D).

**93. D**: Although babies must be fed to survive and crying communicates hunger, babies also cry to meet other needs necessary to their survival; therefore, (A) is untrue. For example, a classic study in the early 1900s found that when infants had only their physical needs met by being fed, changed, bathed, etc., but were never held, cuddled, spoken to or sung to, the majority of them actually died. Therefore, crying aids development only when adults respond to it, so (C) is incorrect. Babies cry not only to meet physical needs (B,) but also to stimulate adults to interact with them physically, emotionally, and socially.

**94. D**: Sigmund Freud's psychoanalytic theory of personality focuses on psychosexual development. His stages of development center on different erogenous zones, sexual impulses, and how they are addressed. An example of a personality theory that focuses on archetypal (A) aspects of development is that of Carl Jung. An example of a personality theory focusing on psychogenic (B) needs as aspects of development is that of Henry Murray. An example of a personality theory focusing on psychosocial (C) aspects of development is that of Erik Erikson.

**95. A**: Albert Bandura proposed in his Social Learning Theory that people learn by observing others' behavior and the rewards (or punishments) those behaviors receive; retaining their observations, and then imitating the behaviors they have observed to obtain similar rewards (or avoiding those behaviors to avoid similar punishments). The "learning" part of Bandura's theory is based on Skinner's (B) behavioral learning theory. However, Bandura differed from Skinner by emphasizing the influence of social interactions. Skinner proposed that our behaviors are shaped by their consequences; Bandura proposed that we need not initially experience the behaviors or consequences directly, but can learn vicariously. Kohlberg (C) is best known for proposing a theory of moral development related to Piaget's stages of cognitive development. Vygotsky (D) proposed social influences on learning like Bandura, but put more emphasis on sociocultural factors of interaction, cooperation, collaboration with, and support from more knowledgeable others than on observation and imitation as Bandura did.

**96. B**: Hans Eysenck proposed three universal personality traits. McCrae and Costa proposed the "Big Five" personality traits. Raymond Cattell arrived at a final list of 16 personality traits by applying statistical factor analysis to his preliminary list of 171 traits, which he had reduced from the original list of more than 4,000 individual personality traits proposed by Gordon Allport. (Allport classified all the traits he identified into three main categories of cardinal, central, and secondary traits; but he identified over 4,000 individual traits based on the number of words he found in a dictionary that described separate personality characteristics.)

**97. C**: The medical model is an older H&HS model. It views the TR client as a patient with an illness that needs to be cured or treated. Thus, treatment is NOT holistic for the broadest client needs (A), but focused on treating the "illness" or condition while disregarding wider needs of the client as a whole person. In the medical model, TR is guided by the physician's diagnosis and prescription rather than independent of them (B). As the primary therapist, the doctor determines what roles are played by other practitioners, including the RT (C). This model is used most in hospital, physical rehabilitation, and other medical settings rather than community settings (D).

**98. D**: The two most directly opposed of the pairs given are the medical model, which focuses on the illness or condition to be treated rather than on the client as a whole person; vs. the person-centered model, which approaches the client as an individual and considers his or her overall needs. The recovery model has this holistic approach in common with the person-centered model (A). The custodial model is an older approach to providing basic needs (not rehabilitation) for populations in institutions, nursing homes, correctional facilities, and group homes; it is largely being replaced by the long-term care model (B), which aims to sustain the maximum health and wellbeing for chronically disabled populations. As such, these two are more related than opposite. The health promotion or health protection model is basically synonymous with the health and wellness model (C).

**99. C**: The International Statistical Classification of Diseases and Related Health Problems (ICD-10) and the International Classification of Functioning, Disability and Health (ICF) are both members of the World Health Organization (WHO)'s family of international classifications. They are not completely unrelated (A); neither are they nearly the same (B); nor are they mutually exclusive (D). Rather, they complement one another and the WHO encourages their concurrent use. Their main difference is that the ICD-10 classifies health conditions by etiology and diagnosis, while the ICF classifies functioning and disability related to those health conditions.

**100. B**: 2020 Census data reported that the "Some Other Race" category was the second most commonly reported race in the US and that the largest increase from 2010 to 2020 data was in the "Multiple Races" category, which increased from about 3% to over 10% of the total population in 2020.

**101. B**: Experts divide multicultural competencies into four areas: Knowledge, Awareness (aka Beliefs and Attitudes), Skills, and Relationship. Knowing how one's own cultural values and biases influence client interactions falls under the area of Awareness, also called Beliefs and Attitudes. The Knowledge area (A) entails getting/having information, respect, and appreciation regarding other cultures and their differences. The Skills (C) area involves sensitivity to unique behaviors of various groups, culturally appropriate communication skills, and other effective behaviors for interacting with culturally diverse groups. The Relationship (D) area requires the therapist to integrate the other three areas and apply them for developing appropriate, effective therapeutic relationships with diverse clients.

**102. B**: The power structure in a given group in terms of how decisions are made within it (outside of therapist direction) most reflects the group systems concept of which roles are played by different members. The systems concept of coalitions forming within the group (A) would be reflected by which members have formed alliances; whether these alliances are temporary or permanent; and which members have conflicts with each other. The systems concept of group boundaries and whether or not or to what degree they will admit new information (C) would be reflected by something like the criteria for entry into the group. The systems concept of how group members communicate (D) would be reflected by things like where group members focus their attention while participating, and whether communication among members is direct and clear.

**103. D**: Parkinson's disease is the third most common cause of dementia and causes dementia symptoms in at least 30% of patients (A), while Alzheimer's disease is the most common cause of dementia and causes at least 65% of the dementia symptoms among neurodegenerative disorders. Kidney failure or liver failure can also cause dementia symptoms (B), as can traumatic brain injuries (C).

**104. A**: Because Cerebral Palsy causes difficulty with control and coordination of muscular movements, TR should encourage the use of the patient's gross motor skills, which involve the limbs and large muscle movements. TR should encourage use of the patient's residual skills to regain more independence following a spinal cord injury (A). TR can use activities that improve range of motion (ROM) for patients with multiple sclerosis (C). TR should promote movement to maintain the patient's muscle tone in cases of Muscular Dystrophy (D).

**105. C**: Helping heart attack patients to develop healthy lifestyles is included in the role of TR. Proper nutrition, stress management, avoiding tobacco and alcohol, etc. can all prevent future recurrences. The inclusion and degree of physical activity depends on the individual patient's condition: According to the American Heart Association's range of functional limitations, Class I means the patient can engage in physical activity without limits (A); Classes II and III define certain limitations on the patient's physical activity (B); and Class IV means the patient is unable to engage in any physical activity at all (D) without experiencing discomfort.

**106. B**: Polycystic ovary syndrome (PCOS) is classified as an endocrine disorder. Endocrine disorders cause glands in the body to produce too much or too little of specific hormones. PKU (A), hemochromatosis (C), and Cystic Fibrosis (D) are classified as metabolic disorders, wherein the body is impaired or unable in processing specific nutrients. In PKU, copper cannot be processed; in hemochromatosis, it is iron. In Cystic Fibrosis, an inherited genetic defect causes production of a protein that creates sticky, thick mucus, which clogs up the lungs and prevents pancreatic enzymes from processing food for proper absorption.

**107. C**: Insects can carry all these types of diseases. For example, malaria is caused by a parasite (A) that is transmitted to humans by mosquitoes. Lyme disease is caused by a bacterium (B) which deer ticks can carry and transmit to humans. The West Nile virus (D) is also commonly transmitted to humans by mosquito bites.

**108. C**: According to the American Speech-Language-Hearing Association (ASHA), normal hearing is measured audiologically as from -10 to 15 decibels (dB) in the better ear (unaided). A loss of 16-25 dB is defined as a slight hearing loss. A mild (A) hearing loss is a loss of 26-40 dB in the better ear. A moderate (C) loss is a loss of 41-55 dB in the better ear. A loss of 56-70 dB is labeled moderately severe. A severe (B) loss is a loss of 71-90 dB in the better ear. A hearing loss in the better ear of 91 dB or more is classified as a profound hearing loss.

**109. A**: A person can be considered legally blind and may still have enough residual vision to be able to see light, shapes, colors, and objects, although not clearly. More severe degrees of visual impairment can mean a legally blind individual can only tell light from dark (B) or can see light and shapes but not colors (C). However, (A) meets the definition of legal blindness, which equals central visual acuity of 20/200 or worse in the better eye with optimal correction; or a visual field of 20 degrees or less. Someone who cannot see anything (D) is blind rather than just legally blind.

**110. D**: While schizophrenia (A) is better known for causing hallucinations and delusions, bipolar disorder (B) can also cause these symptoms in addition to mood swings between mania and depression. Major depression (C), also called major depressive disorder, can also cause psychotic symptoms in severe cases, including delusions and even hallucinations sometimes. Depending on the classification system, this can be called psychotic depression; major depressive disorder with psychotic symptoms; or simply major depressive disorder or major depression.

**111. B**: The AA and other medical models do view addiction as an illness. While some people think this means it is incurable, it is not. All addictions, including addictions to behaviors like gambling, sex, and eating, involve changes in the brain, and especially addictions to substances. These changes can be reversed through treatments including medications, behavior modification, counseling therapy, exercise, etc. Changes in the brain caused by substance abuse generate intense cravings and make continuing use compulsive; hence it is not true that anyone can avoid or recover from addiction using discipline alone (A). An addict need not "hit rock bottom" to begin recovery (C); recovering is easier when begun earlier in the addiction process, and recovery can begin at any time. People need not initially want to recover for treatment to work (D): addicts can benefit equally whether they enter treatment voluntarily or involuntarily. Resistance often dissipates as cravings are reduced and patients begin thinking more clearly.

**112. B**: Normalization entails exposing people with disabilities to the same opportunities in activities and experiences that other people are routinely exposed to according to the prevalent social and cultural norms. Normalization does not mean trying to make people with disabilities look as normal as possible (A). It does not involve requiring disabled people to engage in normal behaviors (C), but rather altering their environments to allow them chances to have normal life experiences. Encouraging them to interact with people their own age (D) is a definition of age-appropriateness rather than normalization. These two concepts are typically closely related in work with people having disabilities, especially intellectual disabilities; nevertheless, they are not the same.

**113. A**: The Department of Health and Human Services (HHS) is NOT one of the agencies responsible for the standards used to enforce the Architectural Barriers Act (ABA) of 1968. The General Services Administration (B), the US Postal Service (C), and the Department of Defense (D) are the other three agencies in addition to the Department of Housing and Urban Development (HUD) that are responsible for standards used to enforce the ABA.

**114. B**: The United Nations Convention on the Rights of Persons with Disabilities was adopted by international organizations, national governments, human rights institutions, and others over several years. Following ratifications, implementation of this document began in 2009. The Declaration on the Rights of Disabled Persons (A) was made by the General Assembly under the United Nations Charter in 1975. The General Assembly adopted the United Nations' Standard Rules

(C) in 1993. The World Programme of Action concerning Disabled Persons (D) was adopted in 1982.

**115. D**: The Older Americans Act (OAA) was first passed by the US Congress in 1965. The ADA (B) was first passed in 1990. The IDEA (C) was first passed as Public Law 94-142 in 1975, renamed the Individuals with Disabilities Education Act (IDEA) in 1990. Therefore, (A) is incorrect, as no two of these were first enacted in the same year.

**116. D**: The National Council for Therapeutic Recreation Certification (NCTRC), which certifies recreation therapists and verifies RTs' credentials for employers and healthcare agencies, has been recognized by the Centers for Medicare and Medicaid Services or CMS (B) and also maintains ongoing recognition by both the Joint Commission (A) and the Commission for Accreditation of Rehabilitation Facilities or CARF (C).

**117. B**: Lazarus' theory proposes that play and recreation build up energy during leisure time that we can access for our work time. Spencer's Surplus Energy Theory (A) proposes the opposite – that we play during leisure time to burn off excess energy that has built up during work time. In his theory, Stanley Hall used the term recapitulation (C) to describe his proposal that we reenact our ancestors' evolution by passing through stages of growth (animal, savage, nomadic, and tribal). In his theory, Karl Groos proposed that we instinctually practice (D) the same behaviors that animals do (hunting, fighting, playing, and survival) to perfect our skills in each area and to prepare our young for life.

**118. B**: Perceived competence is a person's belief that he or she has the abilities and skills equal to the challenges of engaging in a particular leisure activity. This definition is very similar to the definition of the term self-efficacy, coined by social learning theorist Albert Bandura. Intrinsic motivation (A) refers to an individual's wanting to engage in an activity for the personal rewards of enjoyment, gratification, satisfaction, and/or feelings of achievement rather than doing it because of some external influence, like requirements and/or rewards from others outside oneself. Perceived freedom (C) refers to the individual's freedom to choose and engage in an activity without external barriers to participating, without obligations that interfere, and/or without others' control. Positive affect (D) refers to feelings of happiness and enjoyment which leisure produces, and which are closely related to a sense of choice.

**119. C**: While it may surprise some, a 2005 article found that children in Thailand spent more time watching TV, listening to radio, using the internet, and reading for recreation than American children did. Children in Thailand spent more time in all of these recreational categories than the world average. Children in the USA spent just slightly under the world average of hours per week using the internet for recreation at that time; under 1% less time reading than the world average; and more than the world average for watching TV and listening to radio. Thus, the other choices are all incorrect.

**120. A**: Economists have found through research that over the lifetime, the costs to society of being physically inactive are greater than the costs of smoking tobacco, but less than the costs of heavy drinking; hence (B) is incorrect. Since these are not all equal, (C) is incorrect. Since inactive lifestyles cost society more than smoking and less than heavy drinking, (D) is incorrect.

**121. A**: SOAP is an acronym for Subjective, Objective, Assessment, and Plan. The Assessment (A) part (D) contains the doctor(s)'s medical diagnoses and conclusions based on a review of the data collected. The Subjective (S) part (B) contains a narrative of the patient's presenting problem. The Plan (P) part (C) contains what actions the practitioners involved plan to take for treating the

187

patient. Lab values, vital signs, physical examination findings, and other measurements like height, weight, age, etc. are found in the Objective (O) part (D).

**122. A**: O stands for Objective. This part of SOAP charting is for noting objective facts about a patient, including age, height, and weight as in this example. P stands for Plan. This part is for noting what treatments are planned by health care practitioners (e.g., ordering laboratory tests, prescribing medications, performing procedures, making referrals). A stands for Assessment. This part is where the doctor notes his or her diagnosis, and health care professionals note conclusions based on reviewing the data gathered. S stands for Subjective. This part is for recording the patient's presenting complaint, including onset, quality, severity, modifying factors, additional symptoms, and other providers the patient has seen and other treatments received.

**123. B**: The purpose of developing the FIM was to make measurements and data on disability and rehabilitation results more uniform, because measurement and data in this area had lacked such uniformity for a long time. The FIM was not developed to increase options for ways to measure disability and rehab outcomes (A); to generate larger amounts of data on these (C); or to make such measurement and resulting data more versatile (D). It was to standardize the assessments made and information obtained on disability and rehab results in medical inpatient programs.

**124. D**: The FIM is flexible enough that the user can complete it by conferring with the patient and other involved healthcare professionals (A); by making observations of the patient (B); or by conducting telephone interviews (C).

**125. C**: Rasch analysis of the FIM has identified motor (A) and cognitive (B) dimensions of the FIM, but this instrument does not include a psychosocial (D) dimension.

**126. A**: Measurable objectives for a patient care plan should include how progress will be measured (i.e., what instruments will be used?); however, objectives stating the patient will "understand," "appreciate," or "be aware of" anything should be avoided because these terms are not quantifiable (measurable), and are not specific enough to prevent multiple and varying interpretations. Measurable objectives should also specify the time when results are expected AND the criteria to be used for judging successful outcomes (B); which specific outcomes are desired AND how they are to be measured (C). Therefore, BOTH the criteria for identifying success AND the time when it is expected to be accomplished (D) must be included in the objectives.

**127. A**: The US Census figures for 2020 show an increase in time spent doing leisure activities (about 30 minutes more each day) from 2019 due to the lock downs decreasing school and work hours. The most common leisure activity in 2020 was watching tv, while leisure activities such as playing sports decreased due to limitations on group sports during the COVID outbreak.

**128. C**: The greatest emphasis in selecting TR activities for clients recently has been on producing measurable outcomes for them. Experts note that simply providing them with activities (A) is no longer sufficient for RT practice to become a central part of health and human services; stopping short at activity provision will only keep RT at the periphery. This drive toward changing some aspects of client behaviors also means that third-party providers will not reimburse TR charges if activities chosen only offer entertainment without changing behaviors (B). Since the most emphasis is on (C), (D) is incorrect.

**129. C**: Although of course clients should be able to understand the TR activities selected for them by the RT, intelligibility is not a term or concept used in association with activity task analysis or selection. Activities should be relevant, somewhat familiar, and enjoyable to clients. Moreover, three important concepts that TR experts say should guide RTs in selecting activities are causality

(A), meaning that client participation in a selected activity should be very likely to cause the desired outcome (goal); predictability (D), meaning one can reasonably predict the desired outcome from client participation in the activity; and replicability (B), meaning the results can be reproduced: the desired outcome is likely for all or most clients participating in a selected program or activity.

**130. A**: It is true that people with spinal cord injuries can even water-ski: modifications include a special ski with a seat, similar to a toboggan or a sit-ski used in downhill snow skiing, and outriggers to pull the water-skier behind the speedboat. Recreation Departments like that of the City of San Diego or Phoenix, Arizona's Saint Joseph Hospital provide information on adapted water-skiing. It is not true that no group exists to teach scuba diving to the disabled (B): The Handicapped Scuba Association, for example, does train persons with disabilities in scuba diving. It is also not true that no modifications exist for sailing by the disabled (C): sailboats can be modified to permit easier boarding and de-boarding by the disabled, for example. Several groups, including the US Yacht Racing Union and the National Ocean Access Project, help people with disabilities to sail. People with spinal cord injuries can row, but they may need slight adaptations like devices for their arms, so it is not true that they need none (D).

**131. C**: The characteristics of the client described indicate that assertiveness training would meet the client goals of initiating group activities and improving leadership behaviors. Leisure skill development (A) is not indicated as the client is described as knowing how to perform many different leisure activities. Training for social skills (B) is not indicated as the client is described as cooperating and interacting well with others. Stress management (D) is not most indicated because there is no information in the description whether the client is experiencing more stress than is normal or not.

**132. B**: The leisure education that RTs can provide to patients who have become disabled through injuries includes teaching them how to self-advocate. Even people who had good problem-solving skills prior to their injuries may need to be taught new problem-solving skills (A) that are unique to having disabilities. RTs can teach patients their legal disability rights, and also how to cope with discrimination (C) from others. They can teach them not only how to manage their time and energy after becoming disabled, but also how to manage issues related to adjustment (D).

**133. C**: Nobody should ever be excluded from recreation and leisure activities on the basis of their race or ethnicity (A), gender or sexual orientation (B), OR medical history, or employment status (D). While medical history must be considered when designing activities that are safe, appropriate, and possible for the person(s) involved to perform, this does NOT mean it is ever necessary to exclude any of them from recreational and leisure activities.

**134. D**: These are all progressively more behavioral and specific components of the TR program design. The TPO (A) contains general statements of the results that the RT expects the client to accomplish, such as being able to demonstrate knowledge of taking turns. The EOs (C) are smaller segments of behavior contained within the TPO, like demonstrating the ability to take turns with others in group activities. The PMs (B) are behavioral objectives the RT expects the client to attain through program participation. For example: once the client has completed the program, he or she will demonstrate taking turns as shown by the CPDs, which would be stated for each program (e.g., waiting until someone else is finished before taking a turn, taking only one turn at a time, taking a turn when nobody else is).

**135. B**: Health Services are most often combined with Human Services in government agencies because the Federal government, as well as many State and County governments, have Departments of Health and Human Services (HHS). Government agencies do not commonly combine Leisure Services and Health Services (A), Human Services and Education Services (C), or Education Services and Leisure Services (D) in one department. They usually have a separate Department of Education. Leisure services are often included within other departments (e.g., Departments of Parks and Recreation or Departments of Parks, Recreation, and Tourism Services).

**136. B**: Physical therapists (PTs) are likely to work with RTs on the level of the interdisciplinary team. Occupational therapists (OTs), music therapists, and art therapists are more likely to work with RTs not only on the interdisciplinary team level, but also on the levels of developing programs for clients, implementing programs and delivering services, and daily planning.

**137. C**: The PPS is a system of payment for health care services that is based on price. The prices are established in advance of providing services, not after service delivery (A). The prices established DO include all of the services that will be provided (B). Once prices have been established, they are not affected by the actual service costs for the current year (C). Only established prices are charged, and no additional settlements or payments can be assessed (D).

**138. A**: One reason that accurate documentation is important is that the information documented supplies researchers investigating program/treatment efficacy with data, and also furnishes data needed for quality improvement processes. Another reason accurate documentation is important is for ensuring that quality services are delivered (B). An additional reason is that accurate documents make it easier for various staff members to communicate with one another (C). One more reason for the importance of documenting information accurately is to ensure compliance with administrative requirements (D).

**139. B**: Evaluation of TR/RT programs can help keep their practitioners accountable to the donors who finance or support the programs. Program evaluation also does guide the decisions made regarding service delivery and program management (A). It helps practitioners and administrators to assess how effective the program is (C) in accomplishing what it is intended to accomplish. And program evaluation also informs and improves the design of future programs (D) by showing what has and has not worked in the current programs, and helping practitioners to learn more from what they have done.

**140. A**: Decreasing the anxieties of agency administrators and personnel about a potential loss and meeting the agency's legal obligations are classified as pre-loss risk management objectives as they can be done before an anticipated loss actually occurs. Ensuring that the agency survives and continues to operate (B), stabilizing agency earnings and promoting continuing agency growth (C), and minimizing the impact of a loss on other people and society (D) are all classified as post-loss risk management objectives as these must be done following the occurrence of a loss.

**141. D**: The analysis of the community, clients, agency, and TR department helps planners to discover client needs, including those related to licensure; and to develop a mission statement and goals. The conceptualization is the stage of developing the mission statement and comprehensive program goals. The mission statement itself is usually a concise sentence that states the comprehensive RT program's purpose; it serves as the center wherefrom the comprehensive RT program develops. The comprehensive program goals more specifically characterize aspects of the mission statement. These goals are statements of the program developers' intentions rather than directly measurable objectives.

**142. B**: The NCTRC requires an internship to consist of not less than 20 hours a week but not more than 45 hours a week; therefore, (A) is incorrect. The NCTRC also requires the internship to be completed all at only one agency; therefore, (C) is incorrect. NCTRC requirements also include that the internship last for at least 14 consecutive weeks and/or 560 hours; therefore, (D) is incorrect.

**143. D**: One result of the establishment of managed care systems relative to payments for TR services has been that whereas the RTs/RT agencies formerly had the authority for determining the TR service needs of a patient as service providers (C), managed care moved the authority for deciding what TR service needs a patient had to the insurers or HMOs as the payers. Therefore, it is incorrect that managed care has not affected who determines and justifies service needs (A). Since the advent of the managed care model, TRS providers have more often had to justify why their services are needed, rather than no longer having to do so (B).

**144. B**: Accessibility standards for TR/RT facilities and equipment dictate that curb ramps at facilities have grades not exceeding 8.33%, that ramps that are not at curbs have maximum grades of 5%, and that all ramps be in usable condition. Accessibility standards are NOT the same for all recreation areas (e.g., trails and paths are different from playgrounds, and each of these also differs from swimming pools, so the standards for access differ accordingly). Accessibility standards DO mention signs (e.g., they specify that facility signs should have dark-colored backgrounds and light-colored lettering). Accessibility standards also specify that parking spaces should allow at least 12.5 ft by 20.5 ft.

**145. D**: Historically, a number of factors contributed relatively equally to the emergence of TR as a field within health care services. Not only did movements to reform the medical and health care fields promote the growth of TR; but social reform movements also recognized the role of leisure and recreation (A). During World Wars I and II, the development of military hospitals contributed; and the proliferation of public hospitals, private hospitals, and specialty clinics contributed (B) to the growth of TR services and programs. Between 1850 and 1920, the Playground Movement (C) also stimulated the development of programming and services in the field of recreation overall.

**146. A**: The NCTRC academic requirements for the CTRS certification include 18 semester hours at an accredited college or university, with 15 of them being in TR and the rest in Recreation. Prior to 2013, the requirement was previously 12 hours in TR and the rest in Recreation (B). For the CTRS, the NCTRC also requires 18 additional semester hours of supportive courses, including anatomy and physiology, human services, human lifespan growth and development, AND abnormal psychology (C). This certification requires EITHER a major in TR, OR a major in Recreation with an option in TR; either one is permitted (D).

**147. B**: RTs in clinical settings have a significant duty to advocate for people with disabilities following their discharge from health care facilities for their participation and integration in the community, particularly via recreation. Such advocacy includes transportation resources (A), limited knowledge of recreational opportunities (B), lack of access to some facilities (C), and obstacles presented by some people's attitudes toward the disabled (D).

**148. A**: Principle 9, Competence, of the ATRA Code of Ethics states that TR professionals are responsible always to seek to expand their knowledge of TR/RT practice (A). Therefore, competence is included in this code of ethics and (D) is incorrect.

**149. A**: Autism spectrum disorders are classified as developmental disabilities. The RT who wants to provide TRS to autistic individuals can obtain a specialty certification from the NCTRC in this area. NCTRC also offers specialty certification in behavioral health services (B), for providing TRS to individuals diagnosed with mental illnesses and disorders; in community inclusion services (C), for providing TRS to individuals having various disabilities to support their living independently in the community; in physical medicine/rehabilitation (D), for providing TRS to individuals in the treatment of injuries and illnesses that are physically disabling and/or affect movement; and in geriatrics, for providing TRS to elderly individuals.

**150. A**: The NCTRC requires internship supervisors to expose interns to all of the task areas identified in its Job Analysis, not just most (B) or some (C) of them. Exposing the intern to none (D) of the task areas of the NCTRC Job Analysis would constitute a complete failure of supervision and internship. NCTRC particularly emphasizes that the intern must be exposed to all of the Job Analysis Task Areas.

# How to Overcome Test Anxiety

Just the thought of taking a test is enough to make most people a little nervous. A test is an important event that can have a long-term impact on your future, so it's important to take it seriously and it's natural to feel anxious about performing well. But just because anxiety is normal, that doesn't mean that it's helpful in test taking, or that you should simply accept it as part of your life. Anxiety can have a variety of effects. These effects can be mild, like making you feel slightly nervous, or severe, like blocking your ability to focus or remember even a simple detail.

If you experience test anxiety—whether severe or mild—it's important to know how to beat it. To discover this, first you need to understand what causes test anxiety.

## Causes of Test Anxiety

While we often think of anxiety as an uncontrollable emotional state, it can actually be caused by simple, practical things. One of the most common causes of test anxiety is that a person does not feel adequately prepared for their test. This feeling can be the result of many different issues such as poor study habits or lack of organization, but the most common culprit is time management. Starting to study too late, failing to organize your study time to cover all of the material, or being distracted while you study will mean that you're not well prepared for the test. This may lead to cramming the night before, which will cause you to be physically and mentally exhausted for the test. Poor time management also contributes to feelings of stress, fear, and hopelessness as you realize you are not well prepared but don't know what to do about it.

Other times, test anxiety is not related to your preparation for the test but comes from unresolved fear. This may be a past failure on a test, or poor performance on tests in general. It may come from comparing yourself to others who seem to be performing better or from the stress of living up to expectations. Anxiety may be driven by fears of the future—how failure on this test would affect your educational and career goals. These fears are often completely irrational, but they can still negatively impact your test performance.

## Elements of Test Anxiety

As mentioned earlier, test anxiety is considered to be an emotional state, but it has physical and mental components as well. Sometimes you may not even realize that you are suffering from test anxiety until you notice the physical symptoms. These can include trembling hands, rapid heartbeat, sweating, nausea, and tense muscles. Extreme anxiety may lead to fainting or vomiting. Obviously, any of these symptoms can have a negative impact on testing. It is important to recognize them as soon as they begin to occur so that you can address the problem before it damages your performance.

The mental components of test anxiety include trouble focusing and inability to remember learned information. During a test, your mind is on high alert, which can help you recall information and stay focused for an extended period of time. However, anxiety interferes with your mind's natural processes, causing you to blank out, even on the questions you know well. The strain of testing during anxiety makes it difficult to stay focused, especially on a test that may take several hours. Extreme anxiety can take a huge mental toll, making it difficult not only to recall test information but even to understand the test questions or pull your thoughts together.

193

# Effects of Test Anxiety

Test anxiety is like a disease—if left untreated, it will get progressively worse. Anxiety leads to poor performance, and this reinforces the feelings of fear and failure, which in turn lead to poor performances on subsequent tests. It can grow from a mild nervousness to a crippling condition. If allowed to progress, test anxiety can have a big impact on your schooling, and consequently on your future.

Test anxiety can spread to other parts of your life. Anxiety on tests can become anxiety in any stressful situation, and blanking on a test can turn into panicking in a job situation. But fortunately, you don't have to let anxiety rule your testing and determine your grades. There are a number of relatively simple steps you can take to move past anxiety and function normally on a test and in the rest of life.

# Physical Steps for Beating Test Anxiety

While test anxiety is a serious problem, the good news is that it can be overcome. It doesn't have to control your ability to think and remember information. While it may take time, you can begin taking steps today to beat anxiety.

Just as your first hint that you may be struggling with anxiety comes from the physical symptoms, the first step to treating it is also physical. Rest is crucial for having a clear, strong mind. If you are tired, it is much easier to give in to anxiety. But if you establish good sleep habits, your body and mind will be ready to perform optimally, without the strain of exhaustion. Additionally, sleeping well helps you to retain information better, so you're more likely to recall the answers when you see the test questions.

Getting good sleep means more than going to bed on time. It's important to allow your brain time to relax. Take study breaks from time to time so it doesn't get overworked, and don't study right before bed. Take time to rest your mind before trying to rest your body, or you may find it difficult to fall asleep.

Along with sleep, other aspects of physical health are important in preparing for a test. Good nutrition is vital for good brain function. Sugary foods and drinks may give a burst of energy but this burst is followed by a crash, both physically and emotionally. Instead, fuel your body with protein and vitamin-rich foods.

Also, drink plenty of water. Dehydration can lead to headaches and exhaustion, especially if your brain is already under stress from the rigors of the test. Particularly if your test is a long one, drink water during the breaks. And if possible, take an energy-boosting snack to eat between sections.

Along with sleep and diet, a third important part of physical health is exercise. Maintaining a steady workout schedule is helpful, but even taking 5-minute study breaks to walk can help get your blood pumping faster and clear your head. Exercise also releases endorphins, which contribute to a positive feeling and can help combat test anxiety.

When you nurture your physical health, you are also contributing to your mental health. If your body is healthy, your mind is much more likely to be healthy as well. So take time to rest, nourish your body with healthy food and water, and get moving as much as possible. Taking these physical steps will make you stronger and more able to take the mental steps necessary to overcome test anxiety.

# Mental Steps for Beating Test Anxiety

Working on the mental side of test anxiety can be more challenging, but as with the physical side, there are clear steps you can take to overcome it. As mentioned earlier, test anxiety often stems from lack of preparation, so the obvious solution is to prepare for the test. Effective studying may be the most important weapon you have for beating test anxiety, but you can and should employ several other mental tools to combat fear.

First, boost your confidence by reminding yourself of past success—tests or projects that you aced. If you're putting as much effort into preparing for this test as you did for those, there's no reason you should expect to fail here. Work hard to prepare; then trust your preparation.

Second, surround yourself with encouraging people. It can be helpful to find a study group, but be sure that the people you're around will encourage a positive attitude. If you spend time with others who are anxious or cynical, this will only contribute to your own anxiety. Look for others who are motivated to study hard from a desire to succeed, not from a fear of failure.

Third, reward yourself. A test is physically and mentally tiring, even without anxiety, and it can be helpful to have something to look forward to. Plan an activity following the test, regardless of the outcome, such as going to a movie or getting ice cream.

When you are taking the test, if you find yourself beginning to feel anxious, remind yourself that you know the material. Visualize successfully completing the test. Then take a few deep, relaxing breaths and return to it. Work through the questions carefully but with confidence, knowing that you are capable of succeeding.

Developing a healthy mental approach to test taking will also aid in other areas of life. Test anxiety affects more than just the actual test—it can be damaging to your mental health and even contribute to depression. It's important to beat test anxiety before it becomes a problem for more than testing.

# Study Strategy

Being prepared for the test is necessary to combat anxiety, but what does being prepared look like? You may study for hours on end and still not feel prepared. What you need is a strategy for test prep. The next few pages outline our recommended steps to help you plan out and conquer the challenge of preparation.

## STEP 1: SCOPE OUT THE TEST

Learn everything you can about the format (multiple choice, essay, etc.) and what will be on the test. Gather any study materials, course outlines, or sample exams that may be available. Not only will this help you to prepare, but knowing what to expect can help to alleviate test anxiety.

## STEP 2: MAP OUT THE MATERIAL

Look through the textbook or study guide and make note of how many chapters or sections it has. Then divide these over the time you have. For example, if a book has 15 chapters and you have five days to study, you need to cover three chapters each day. Even better, if you have the time, leave an extra day at the end for overall review after you have gone through the material in depth.

If time is limited, you may need to prioritize the material. Look through it and make note of which sections you think you already have a good grasp on, and which need review. While you are studying, skim quickly through the familiar sections and take more time on the challenging parts.

Write out your plan so you don't get lost as you go. Having a written plan also helps you feel more in control of the study, so anxiety is less likely to arise from feeling overwhelmed at the amount to cover.

## STEP 3: GATHER YOUR TOOLS

Decide what study method works best for you. Do you prefer to highlight in the book as you study and then go back over the highlighted portions? Or do you type out notes of the important information? Or is it helpful to make flashcards that you can carry with you? Assemble the pens, index cards, highlighters, post-it notes, and any other materials you may need so you won't be distracted by getting up to find things while you study.

If you're having a hard time retaining the information or organizing your notes, experiment with different methods. For example, try color-coding by subject with colored pens, highlighters, or post-it notes. If you learn better by hearing, try recording yourself reading your notes so you can listen while in the car, working out, or simply sitting at your desk. Ask a friend to quiz you from your flashcards, or try teaching someone the material to solidify it in your mind.

## STEP 4: CREATE YOUR ENVIRONMENT

It's important to avoid distractions while you study. This includes both the obvious distractions like visitors and the subtle distractions like an uncomfortable chair (or a too-comfortable couch that makes you want to fall asleep). Set up the best study environment possible: good lighting and a comfortable work area. If background music helps you focus, you may want to turn it on, but otherwise keep the room quiet. If you are using a computer to take notes, be sure you don't have any other windows open, especially applications like social media, games, or anything else that could distract you. Silence your phone and turn off notifications. Be sure to keep water close by so you stay hydrated while you study (but avoid unhealthy drinks and snacks).

Also, take into account the best time of day to study. Are you freshest first thing in the morning? Try to set aside some time then to work through the material. Is your mind clearer in the afternoon or evening? Schedule your study session then. Another method is to study at the same time of day that you will take the test, so that your brain gets used to working on the material at that time and will be ready to focus at test time.

## STEP 5: STUDY!

Once you have done all the study preparation, it's time to settle into the actual studying. Sit down, take a few moments to settle your mind so you can focus, and begin to follow your study plan. Don't give in to distractions or let yourself procrastinate. This is your time to prepare so you'll be ready to fearlessly approach the test. Make the most of the time and stay focused.

Of course, you don't want to burn out. If you study too long you may find that you're not retaining the information very well. Take regular study breaks. For example, taking five minutes out of every hour to walk briskly, breathing deeply and swinging your arms, can help your mind stay fresh.

As you get to the end of each chapter or section, it's a good idea to do a quick review. Remind yourself of what you learned and work on any difficult parts. When you feel that you've mastered the material, move on to the next part. At the end of your study session, briefly skim through your notes again.

But while review is helpful, cramming last minute is NOT. If at all possible, work ahead so that you won't need to fit all your study into the last day. Cramming overloads your brain with more information than it can process and retain, and your tired mind may struggle to recall even previously learned information when it is overwhelmed with last-minute study. Also, the urgent nature of cramming and the stress placed on your brain contribute to anxiety. You'll be more likely to go to the test feeling unprepared and having trouble thinking clearly.

So don't cram, and don't stay up late before the test, even just to review your notes at a leisurely pace. Your brain needs rest more than it needs to go over the information again. In fact, plan to finish your studies by noon or early afternoon the day before the test. Give your brain the rest of the day to relax or focus on other things, and get a good night's sleep. Then you will be fresh for the test and better able to recall what you've studied.

## STEP 6: TAKE A PRACTICE TEST

Many courses offer sample tests, either online or in the study materials. This is an excellent resource to check whether you have mastered the material, as well as to prepare for the test format and environment.

Check the test format ahead of time: the number of questions, the type (multiple choice, free response, etc.), and the time limit. Then create a plan for working through them. For example, if you have 30 minutes to take a 60-question test, your limit is 30 seconds per question. Spend less time on the questions you know well so that you can take more time on the difficult ones.

If you have time to take several practice tests, take the first one open book, with no time limit. Work through the questions at your own pace and make sure you fully understand them. Gradually work up to taking a test under test conditions: sit at a desk with all study materials put away and set a timer. Pace yourself to make sure you finish the test with time to spare and go back to check your answers if you have time.

After each test, check your answers. On the questions you missed, be sure you understand why you missed them. Did you misread the question (tests can use tricky wording)? Did you forget the information? Or was it something you hadn't learned? Go back and study any shaky areas that the practice tests reveal.

Taking these tests not only helps with your grade, but also aids in combating test anxiety. If you're already used to the test conditions, you're less likely to worry about it, and working through tests until you're scoring well gives you a confidence boost. Go through the practice tests until you feel comfortable, and then you can go into the test knowing that you're ready for it.

## Test Tips

On test day, you should be confident, knowing that you've prepared well and are ready to answer the questions. But aside from preparation, there are several test day strategies you can employ to maximize your performance.

First, as stated before, get a good night's sleep the night before the test (and for several nights before that, if possible). Go into the test with a fresh, alert mind rather than staying up late to study.

Try not to change too much about your normal routine on the day of the test. It's important to eat a nutritious breakfast, but if you normally don't eat breakfast at all, consider eating just a protein bar. If you're a coffee drinker, go ahead and have your normal coffee. Just make sure you time it so that the caffeine doesn't wear off right in the middle of your test. Avoid sugary beverages, and drink enough water to stay hydrated but not so much that you need a restroom break 10 minutes into the test. If your test isn't first thing in the morning, consider going for a walk or doing a light workout before the test to get your blood flowing.

Allow yourself enough time to get ready, and leave for the test with plenty of time to spare so you won't have the anxiety of scrambling to arrive in time. Another reason to be early is to select a good seat. It's helpful to sit away from doors and windows, which can be distracting. Find a good seat, get out your supplies, and settle your mind before the test begins.

When the test begins, start by going over the instructions carefully, even if you already know what to expect. Make sure you avoid any careless mistakes by following the directions.

Then begin working through the questions, pacing yourself as you've practiced. If you're not sure on an answer, don't spend too much time on it, and don't let it shake your confidence. Either skip it and come back later, or eliminate as many wrong answers as possible and guess among the remaining ones. Don't dwell on these questions as you continue—put them out of your mind and focus on what lies ahead.

Be sure to read all of the answer choices, even if you're sure the first one is the right answer. Sometimes you'll find a better one if you keep reading. But don't second-guess yourself if you do immediately know the answer. Your gut instinct is usually right. Don't let test anxiety rob you of the information you know.

If you have time at the end of the test (and if the test format allows), go back and review your answers. Be cautious about changing any, since your first instinct tends to be correct, but make sure you didn't misread any of the questions or accidentally mark the wrong answer choice. Look over any you skipped and make an educated guess.

At the end, leave the test feeling confident. You've done your best, so don't waste time worrying about your performance or wishing you could change anything. Instead, celebrate the successful completion of this test. And finally, use this test to learn how to deal with anxiety even better next time.

> **Review Video: Test Anxiety**
> Visit mometrix.com/academy and enter code: 100340

## Important Qualification

Not all anxiety is created equal. If your test anxiety is causing major issues in your life beyond the classroom or testing center, or if you are experiencing troubling physical symptoms related to your anxiety, it may be a sign of a serious physiological or psychological condition. If this sounds like your situation, we strongly encourage you to seek professional help.

# Online Resources

Due to our efforts to try to keep this book to a manageable length, we've created a link that will give you access to all of your online resources:

**mometrix.com/resources719/nctrc**

# It's Your Moment, Let's Celebrate It!

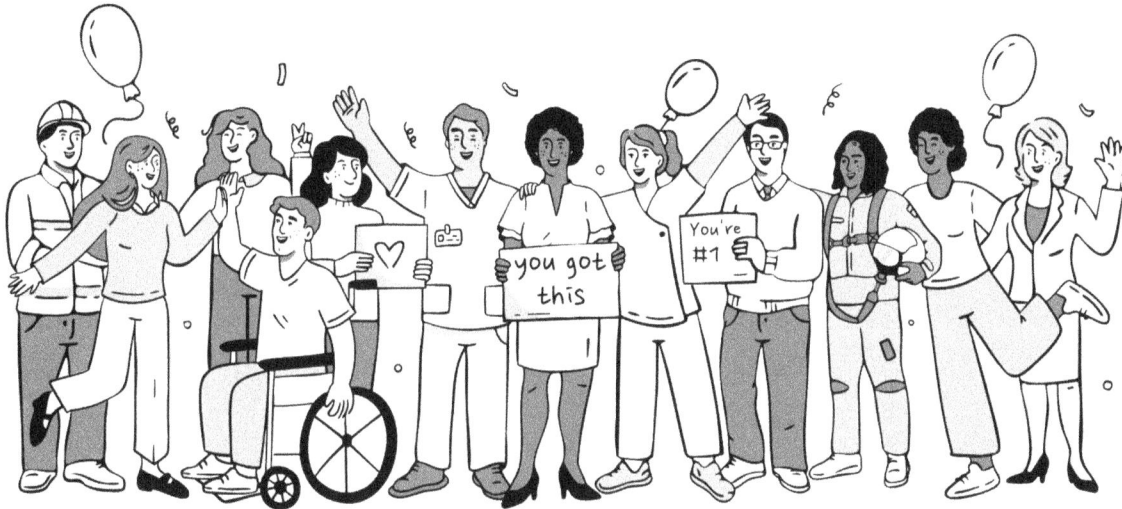

**Share your story @mometrixtestpreparation**